UNAGING

Aging is a subject of concern to everyone, but is widely misunderstood. If we view it as inevitable, we miss the fact that not everyone is able to grow to an old age. Realization of this reality helps us to understand that aging presents a wonderful opportunity – an opportunity to make choices about how we live which can enhance the aging process and offer a chance to live to our potential.

This book clearly presents the four reserve factors (cognitive, physical, psychological, and social) which impact our ability to have healthy responses to the stresses of aging. By giving the biological basis for the advice given, you will learn the steps to take in your activities, diet, and mental outlook to grasp the opportunity that aging offers. Everyone must know that what we do makes a difference.

Robert Friedland MD is a neurologist and the Rudd endowed professor of Neurology and Neurobiology at the University of Louisville School of Medicine in Kentucky. He previously worked at the University of California, Berkeley, the US National Institute on Aging, and Case Western Reserve University. Recently his research has uncovered a key role of intestinal bacteria in the initiation and progression of Alzheimer's disease, Parkinson's disease, and amyotrophic lateral sclerosis. His studies of humans and animals in the United States, Japan, the Middle East, and Kenya have helped to advance the concept that the risk of aging-related brain diseases can be lowered through our personal actions.

"Rooted on his vast clinical and research experience, Dr. Friedland takes us on an accessible scientific tour to demystify the inevitability of aging. Dementia, he highlights with a wealth of examples, is not preordained in anyone, even in individuals with high-risk genetic mutations or with brain amyloid plaques. Dr. Friedland reviews the evidence accumulated to make his case that specific changes in our own environment can shape how we age – or not."

Alberto Espay, author of *Brain Fables: The Hidden History of Neurodegenerative Diseases and a Blueprint to Conquer Them*

"Dr. Friedland's idea that aging is not inevitable is not fully recognized by the general public. However, recent advances in geriatrics show that his idea 'aging is not inevitable' is correct. This book is impressive because he teaches us the mechanisms of aging and how to enhance aging. It's possible to change your life from this book. I hope you will know the truth and gain a wonderful tool against aging."

Professor Toshiki Mizuno, Kyoto Prefectural University of Medicine

"In his book, *Unaging*, Dr. Friedland begins by setting the stage, describing the importance of physical, mental, psychological, and social health, and explaining that the goal is not normal aging, but exceptional aging. He then teaches you how to attack and subdue the harmful habits that accelerate aging by extrapolating the results of rigorous scientific studies. This book is a 'must read' for anyone who would like to use the latest scientific studies to help them live healthier lives as they age."

Andrew E. Budson, author of *Seven Steps to Managing Your Memory: What's Normal, What's Not, and What to Do About It*

"You have to grow old but you don't have to age. This is the book that tells you how to do it."

Nori Graham, author of *A Pocket Guide to Understanding Alzheimer's Disease and Other Dementias*

"With clear language and an attention-grabbing narrative style, Dr. Friedland introduces and discusses many of the issues related to aging that represent the pillars of the science on the subject. From an original perspective, the book addresses the so-called reserve factors, neurological diseases, mental health, and most importantly, the actions we need to take to improve our chances of a healthy and satisfactory aging, where aging is seen as a blessing, not as a burden. The book closes with the chapter 'The opportunity of aging' which, in my interpretation, summarizes the author's overview.

Anyone interested in aging should read this text."

Dr. Carmen García Peña, *Instituto Nacional de Geriatría*

Unaging

The Four Factors that Impact How You Age

ROBERT P. FRIEDLAND

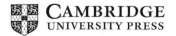
CAMBRIDGE
UNIVERSITY PRESS

CAMBRIDGE
UNIVERSITY PRESS

University Printing House, Cambridge CB2 8BS, United Kingdom

One Liberty Plaza, 20th Floor, New York, NY 10006, USA

477 Williamstown Road, Port Melbourne, VIC 3207, Australia

314–321, 3rd Floor, Plot 3, Splendor Forum, Jasola District Centre, New Delhi – 110025, India

103 Penang Road, #05–06/07, Visioncrest Commercial, Singapore 238467

Cambridge University Press is part of the University of Cambridge.

It furthers the University's mission by disseminating knowledge in the pursuit of education, learning, and research at the highest international levels of excellence.

www.cambridge.org
Information on this title: www.cambridge.org/9781009087742
DOI: 10.1017/9781009083645

© Cambridge University Press 2022

First published 2022

A catalogue record for this publication is available from the British Library.

Library of Congress Cataloging-in-Publication Data
Names: Friedland, Robert P., author.
Title: Unaging : the four factors that impact how you age / Robert P Friedland.
Description: Cambridge, United Kingdom ; New York, NY : Cambridge University Press, 2022. | Includes bibliographical references and index.
Identifiers: LCCN 2021063076 (print) | LCCN 2021063077 (ebook) | ISBN 9781009087742 (paperback) | ISBN 9781009083645 (ebook)
Subjects: LCSH: Aging–Prevention. | Older people–Health and hygiene. | Longevity. | Quality of life. | BISAC: HEALTH & FITNESS / Longevity
Classification: LCC RA776.75 .F74 2022 (print) | LCC RA776.75 (ebook) | DDC 613.2–dc23/eng/20220211
LC record available at https://lccn.loc.gov/2021063076
LC ebook record available at https://lccn.loc.gov/2021063077

ISBN 978-1-009-08774-2 Paperback

To my patients and their current and future families.

CONTENTS

List of figures and tables   *page* x
Preface   xi

**PART I FOUNDATIONS: WHAT DO WE NEED
         TO KNOW ABOUT OPTIMAL AGING?**   1

1 AGING IS NOT INEVITABLE, IT IS AN
  OPPORTUNITY   3

2 THE THEORY OF THE MULTIPLE RESERVE
  FACTORS   25

3 THE BRAIN IS NOT AN ORGAN, IT IS THE
  MASTER   42

4 MEMORY AND COGNITION   60

5 THE NEURODEGENERATIVE DISEASES
  OF AGING   76

6 STROKE AND VASCULAR COGNITIVE
  IMPAIRMENT   107

7 OTHER DEMENTIAS   117

8 OUR MICROBIOTA AND HOW TO DO GENE
  THERAPY IN THE KITCHEN   126

9 THE HEALTH OF THE BODY AND THE
  PHYSICAL RESERVE FACTOR   148

10 DEPRESSION, ANXIETY, AND WHAT GOOD
     IS FEELING BAD?   161

11 GENETICS AREN'T EVERYTHING   170

**PART II APPLICATIONS: WHAT CAN WE DO
              ABOUT THE OPPORTUNITY OF AGING? 183**

12 OVERVIEW   185

13 PHYSICAL ACTIVITY   192

14 WHOLE BODY HEALTH   198

15 MENTAL ACTIVITY   200

16 PSYCHOLOGICAL MEASURES   206

17 SOCIAL FACTORS   216

18 DEALING WITH STRESS   219

19 SLEEP   222

20 DIET   225

21 MICROBIAL CONSIDERATIONS   246

22 DENTAL CARE   249

23 DEALING WITH DOCTORS AND DRUGS   250

24 HAZARDOUS BEHAVIORS   269

25 TOXIC EXPOSURES   274

PART III CONCLUSIONS 279

26 CONSIDERATIONS FOR SOCIETY AND THE FUTURE OF AGING 281

27 OUR ATTITUDE AND THE OPPORTUNITY OF AGING 292

Acknowledgments 298
Glossary 300
References 303
Index 320

LIST OF FIGURES
AND TABLES

Figures

1. Declines in function with aging   *page* 14
2. Variability increases with age   15
3. Cognitive reserve factor   27
4. The four reserves and Alzheimer's disease   40
5. Pathways from gut to brain and brain to gut   89
6. Relative odds of Alzheimer's disease according
   to APOE genotype and age in Caucasian subjects   175

Tables

1. Changes with aging in the body and brain   5
2. The three goals of aging   7
3. Diseases and processes influenced
   by the microbiota   129
4. Examples of the influence of the microbiota on
   the body   130

PREFACE

Act as if whatever you do makes a difference. It does.
William James (1842–1910), Harvard University psychologist
and philosopher, author of *Principles of Psychology*

Just about everyone wants to know the secret to a long and healthy life. You may think exercise and mental health are key. Both are important, but in fact there are four factors that are central to vibrant living. The key to successful aging is the maintenance of our bodies' four reserve factors: cognitive, physical, psychological, and social. The status of these reserve factors is a critical component of health and fitness throughout life and is of special importance in aging. Our four reserve factors function to maintain the balance of our body systems, despite the challenges which are encountered. As you will see throughout the book, there are many things we can do to enhance our reserve capacity and preserve our function as we age.

But does it matter what we do? Why should we care? I'd like to tell you why this is important to me, and to you.

As a neurologist, I've spent a lifetime studying how the brain works in health and disease and what can be done to enhance brain health with aging. In this book, I'll reveal what I've learned by explaining and demonstrating the importance of the four reserve factors, which are critical to healthy aging. You see, when we're young, our bodies and brains can handle all sorts of bad behavior, including excessive drinking, lack of sleep, and eating too much junk food. That's because our young bodies have the reserve capacity to keep us going. But as we age, this capacity diminishes and our resilience suffers unless we carefully cultivate and nuture these four reserve factors.

I will tell you more about this and other essential knowledge in a down-to-earth, readable way that will help you understand your brain, body, and what you can do to keep them perky as you age.

The years of life after the sixth decade should be amongst the happiest of all. This is the time when older persons can enjoy retirement, spend time with family, and devote themselves to special interests, without the need for work. Unfortunately, the quality of these years is often tragically damaged by the neurodegenerative diseases associated with aging: Alzheimer's disease, Parkinson's disease, and amyotrophic lateral sclerosis (ALS) (also known as Lou Gehrig's disease), as well as stroke. As a practicing neurologist for the past 45 years, I have been devoted to taking care of these patients and their families.

The central focus of my efforts in patient care and research is to improve the health of older persons, and to understand why people get these conditions and how they can be prevented. Although our knowledge has improved greatly over these five decades, we still don't know why most people are affected. I have pursued this work because our knowledge of these diseases is so poor and the ways to help patients are so limited.

For many years, it has been my mission to proclaim the truth that aging is not inevitable – that what we do makes a difference. I have written this book to clarify my positive approach, that there are many things you can do to improve your prospects with aging. The book begins by presenting the scientific basis of these recommendations and then outlines specific actions that will enhance your brain and body as you age. My aim is to help you understand the most important, and the least understood, part of the body: the brain. I will also explain how the brain interacts with the rest of the body and how our response to aging is influenced by our lifestyle choices.

How can we appreciate the work of the brain and its relation with the body? Consider an ordinary day. When I wake up, I am usually aware of what time it is. Somehow, my brain has calculated the approximate time. I notice the relative temperature of the room and move my legs off the bed and onto the floor, which changes my center of gravity so that I can sit up. Regardless of what I am thinking about, my brain calculates what needs to be done on this ordinary morning. The blood flow to my hands and feet is controlled in a dynamic fashion so that I do not lose too much heat. I go to the kitchen and put two pieces of whole wheat bread in the toaster. The movements necessary for this task are quite complex, considering that they involve muscles in the fingers, wrists, forearms, and shoulders. No matter how complicated the movements, I don't think about them. When the toast pops up, warmed to perfection and crisp, I cover the bread with fig jam, walk to the dining room, sit down, and eat. (Note how both the whole wheat bread and fig jam are both high in fiber, but I am getting ahead of myself.)

At the same time I am waking up and having breakfast, my heart is adapting to the demands made on it, and my liver is delivering glucose to my bloodstream. My liver is also managing the nutrients contained in my breakfast and storing energy as glycogen, and delivering amino acids and other molecules to the rest of my body. My immune system in the gut and elsewhere is monitoring the presence of microbes and microbial products to provide both cellular and antibody defenses against potential pathogens (disease-causing agents). In addition, the microbes in my gut are interacting with my immune system in a way which hopefully limits the development of inflammatory factors that lead to disease. My urinary bladder is monitoring its contents. My brain is busy supervising my blood volume, body temperature, blood pressure, blood sugar, blood sodium content (all critical to life), and evaluating the need for changes in heart rate, cardiac output, tone of blood vessels, sweating, water intake, excretion, and posture.

Thus, in a few moments of an ordinary morning my brain has made multiple complex calculations regarding my well-being. And other parts of my body have also been busy maintaining my health. *We all have the delusion that we are in charge of everything, when actually the most important of human activities are automatic.* As humans, all we can do is oversee the intricate interactions that go on between the brain and other parts of our bodies. The unconscious nature of these actions allows us to survive in a world with myriad stimuli which would overburden our consciousness if we needed to pay attention to every task.

These processes involved in waking up are all interrelated: the brain perceives the body, and the body reacts to the brain. There is no part of us which is truly independent, just as there is no person who is truly independent of others. This state of complex interdependence is found from birth throughout life and is the key to healthy aging. The center of this process is the brain. No wonder the Spanish brain scientist Santiago Ramón y Cajal compared the brain's cerebral cortex to "a garden full of an infinite number of trees." The neurons comprising Cajal's trees are vital entities that change according to interactions with the world and with the body. They grow and adapt like trees in a heavy wind. The trees of the cerebral cortex are changed by how we use them and by their relationship to the rest of our bodies.

The French physiologist Claude Bernard (1813–1878) marveled at how the body regulated itself. He coined the term "milieu interieur" to describe the interactions within the body that produced steadiness and health. He said, "the stability of the internal environment (the "milieu interieur") is the condition for a free and independent life." Bernard, who was a friend of Louis Pasteur, recognized the ability of the brain to compensate for external conditions and maintain the balance of body processes "so that its equilibrium results from a continuous and delicate compensation established as if the most sensitive of balances."[1]

There is a potential danger in Bernard's use of the metaphor of "balances" applied to the "milieu interieur." That is, we have a mental image of a balance having two arms, allowing for the weight of one substance or object to be compared with the weight of another. In reality, our internal processes are supremely complex and multifaceted. All of our body parts are interconnected and interdependent (mutually dependent). The balance of our internal structures involves an innumerable number of variables, such as body temperature, blood pressure, heart rate, circulating concentration of red blood cells and electrolytes (such as sodium, potassium, and chloride), and countless others. Moreover, the interactions at the heart of a balanced body are not limited to forces producing increases or decreases in a variable. Frequently, these manipulations involve modulations in which the excitability and other aspects of an organ and its interactions can be adjusted. A healthy, balanced body involves the equilibrium of all body processes, including responses to stress and maintenance of the body's barriers.

The ability of the body to maintain stability among the interdependent elements we have been discussing is called "homeostasis," which describes the processes that allow for stability of body functions (Walter Cannon popularized the concept of homeostasis in his book *The Wisdom of the Body*, first published in 1932). The word homeostasis comes from "homeo" (similar to) and "stasis" (standing still). Healthy aging requires us to maintain this stability despite the challenges we all face from the stresses we encounter as we age.

Through millions of years of evolution our bodies have evolved the capacity to precisely monitor and adjust themselves in response to internal and external conditions. Although the brain is largely responsible for monitoring the balance of the body's systems, it is heavily dependent on the coordinated functioning of the whole. The brain does not work alone. There are vital interactions of the brain with the circulatory system, gastrointestinal tract, immune responses, and other vital processes. With aging, the quality of these interactions becomes more delicate. The interdependence of our brain with our other organs, as well as the interactions of ourselves with others, is the key to health and fitness with aging.

The interdependence of our brain with our other organs, as well as the interactions of ourselves with others, is the key to health and fitness with aging.

After reading this book, you'll better understand the interactions of the brain, body, physical environment, and society that determine health, disease, fitness, and longevity. The wonderful part of this discussion is that it can lead to actions that enhance quality of life, avoid disease, enhance fitness, and provide meaning with aging.

A chief reason these interactions are not recognized for their critical nature is that the reserve capacity in early life is so high. Young people are very well made and are resilient to damage from unhealthy behaviors. They can often suffer partial losses in function without apparent effect. Because of evolution, young people are frequently able to have poor lifestyle habits which do not notably impact their health. With age, our reserve capacity is reduced and the interdependent interactions we are about to discuss become critical and vital to health and fitness. The concept of reserve capacity comes from the idea of military forces which are "withheld from action to serve as later reinforcements" (OED online). The reserves are ready for activity and available to serve when needed. Similarly, our reserve factors allow us to have resilient responses to challenges which occur in our lives.

The key words here are attention and attitude. As I continue my breakfast, what further dietary choices will I make? Will I be involved in cognitive and physical tasks on this ordinary day? Attention to the role that daily lifestyle choices have in health and fitness is necessary throughout life, and especially important in aging. Will my attitude toward aging be negative, considering it to be uniformly negative? Or will I appreciate the truth that aging is an opportunity to be welcomed with gratitude?

Our recognition of the miracle of our life and function is dependent upon the attitude we have in regard to our survival, and our ability to appreciate the opportunities of aging. *What we do makes a difference.* This book presents detailed advice about what each one of us can do to enhance our experience of aging. Even though we cannot stop all age-related declines in function, we can delay their onset and reduce their impact on our lives.

Robert P. Friedland, M.D.
Louisville, Kentucky

PART I

FOUNDATIONS: WHAT DO WE NEED TO KNOW ABOUT OPTIMAL AGING?

1 AGING IS NOT INEVITABLE, IT IS AN OPPORTUNITY

Our greatest freedom is the freedom to choose our attitude.
Viktor Frankl, Austrian psychiatrist,
author of *Man's Search for Meaning*

A 94-year-old businessman came to see me for an annual check-up. He had been consulting me on a yearly basis for three years and each time had the same complaint. "I am developing Alzheimer's disease," he said. I asked why he thought that he had the disease. His response? "I can't remember who wrote *The Red and the Black*,"[1] he said.

I evaluated him a third time using standard blood tests, and assessment of cognitive functions (tests of memory and reasoning). A year earlier, magnetic resonance imaging of the brain showed some shrinkage of the brain, often seen in healthy people of his age. Memory and cognitive testing showed no decline from the previous year and revealed no significant shortfalls. He also complained of pain in his knees. "When do your knees hurt?" I asked. "When I walk up the four flights to my office," he replied.

At this point I told him that failure to remember the author of *The Red and the Black* was not a sign of Alzheimer's disease. Although I applauded his desire to exercise, I suggested he use the elevator rather than walk up four flights of stairs. I noticed his visits of the previous two years were quite similar to this one, and each time he was concerned about his memory and physical functions. I counseled him

[1] A historical novel of Stendhal, 1830, a French novelist.

as to the effects of age on the brain and the body. I told him that of all the men born 94 years ago in the United States, only 8 percent were still alive, and less than half of those alive still lived independently, and very few of them would have an office and be able to walk up four flights of stairs. It's important for a person to understand the relative nature of his or her position in life.

It's important for a person to understand the relative nature of his or her position in life.

I encouraged him to consider his loss of abilities in the context of his extraordinary survival and overall maintenance of cognitive and physical skills. I told him not to expect his memory to work as well at 94 as it did at 49!

Our response to a situation is heavily affected by our expectations. If the thoughts in anticipation of an event are negative, our perceptions will be biased negatively. If, on the other hand, we have positive expectations, we may be biased in the other direction. Thus, it is critical to consider what our expectations of aging are.

In this chapter we will first consider our expectations and goals for aging and learn what it is that happens as we get older. We will also review the important role of the immune system with aging and how an evolutionary approach helps to inform our choices of actions to improve our aging.

What Are Our Goals for Aging?

As we consider the scenario presented by aging it is important to ask what our expectation are. Do we wish to have normal aging, where the decline in function of all organ systems is accompanied by an increased risk of dying (mortality) and increased risk of disease? Consider what happens with normal aging. Most Americans over the age of 65 years suffer from high blood pressure. And most say they don't have excellent or very good health. On average, people over the age of 65 years have more than two chronic medical conditions. According to the United States Social Security Administration (www.ssa.gov/OACT/TR/2021/index.html), more than 40 percent of people over the age of 75 years have difficulty in physical functioning and 50 percent of people aged 85 years and over need personal assistance with everyday activities. Changes with aging are summarized in Table 1.

The goal isn't "normal aging." The goal is to make terrific choices so you can achieve *exceptional* aging.

I propose three goals for aging (Table 2). The first two are rather obvious, but the third goal is not properly recognized. The first goal of aging is not dying. This is not to deny the inevitability of death, but rather to state the clear truth that most people want to continue living. Most of us want the opportunity to survive from one day to the next. Similarly, we all share the second goal of aging, which is to avoid disease. It's perfectly reasonable that a 30-year-old woman will hope that she can live to be 70 years of age (and more, of course) and, at that older age, she will not have cancer, coronary artery disease, Alzheimer's disease, or other age-related conditions.

Table 1 *Changes with aging in the body and brain*

Decreased
- Recall, reasoning, spatial awareness, speed of perception, and numerical abilities
- Learning and processing speed
- Spatial and working memory
- Size of the brain and density of synapses
- Production of neurotransmitters (especially acetylcholine) involved in memory and learning
- Myelin in the white matter of the brain

Table 1 *(cont.)*

- Speed of impulse transmission in peripheral nerves
- Cerebral blood flow and use of oxygen and glucose
- Serotonin and dopamine receptors
- Visual acuity, depth perception, contrast sensitivity, and dark adaptation
- Vestibular function (balance mechanisms in the ear are less effective)
- Hair cells in the inner ear, cochlear neurons, and high-frequency hearing
- Discrimination of source of sounds and of target from noise
- Vibration sense in feet
- Exercise tolerance
- Pacemaker cells in the heart (more atrial fibrillation)
- Heart relaxation, maximum heart rate
- Sensitivity for blood pressure changes, with increased potential for low blood pressure with posture changes, blood loss or dehydration, fever, sepsis, or medications
- Elastic quality of the lung
- Strength of respiratory muscles and respiratory capacity
- Sex hormones
- Insulin responsiveness
- Regulation of the stress response with delayed recovery
- Ability of the kidney to filter blood and dilute and concentrate the urine (increased risk for dehydration)
- Thirst perception
- Water regulatory capacity
- Total body water
- Muscle mass and strength
- Bone strength
- Maximal oxygen consumption
- Exercise tolerance

Table 1 *(cont.)*

- Gut absorption, contraction, blood flow, and digestive enzyme secretion
- Microbial diversity in the gut

Increased

- Variability of all measures of structure and function
- Toxic misfolded protein collections in the brain
- Inflammation in the blood and brain ("inflammaging")[2]
- Body fat
- Reaction times
- Vocabulary, semantic knowledge (crystalized intelligence, accumulation of knowledge)
- Risk for dehydration and high or low blood sodium levels
- Blood vessel stiffness and risk of hypertension
- Likelihood of falls
- Risk of many diseases of the brain, lungs, heart, blood, gastrointestinal tract, circulation, skin, and other organs

Table 2 *The three goals of aging*

1. Not dying (survival)
2. Not being ill (not having disease)
3. Being fit (enhancing and maintaining function, having strong cognitive, physical, psychological, and social reserves)

Let's add another dimension to these goals to allow ourselves to age exceptionally.

The third goal for aging must be the maintenance of high levels of function (fitness) into later ages, as well as continued well-being and resistance to loss of function.

The third goal for aging must be the maintenance of high levels of function (fitness) into later ages, as well as continued well-being and resistance to loss of function. Imagine two 70-year-old people who have both met the first two goals of aging (that is, they have survived to the age of 70 and have not developed disease conditions of note). However, one may not be able to walk more than a short distance without hip pain and shortness of breath, is no longer able to play golf or swim, has diminished exercise tolerance, and has a lowered resistance to the damaging effects of stress. The other 70-year-old is physically fit and happily participating in meaningful activities, with good abilities to resist stressors. We are all confronted with physical and psychological challenges as we get older. The ability to survive and prosper despite these challenges is a critical factor in aging.

Persons concerned about quality of life with aging must consider all three goals. How can they achieve the three goals of an active, healthy, and long life? That is, what can they do enhance their chance of a long life, free of disease? Equally importantly, they need to ask what they can do to increase the likelihood that they will have the highest level of fitness and resilience (resistance to loss of function) as they age. Resistance to loss of function can also be called reserve capacity. This book presents the theory of multiple reserves (Chapter 2), which examines the concept of the four reserve factors: cognitive, physical, psychological, and social, all of which are key to successfully meeting the three goals of aging.

Avoiding death and sickness is desirable, but it is not enough.

Avoiding death and sickness is desirable, but it is not enough. Just ask the Struldbruggs. In Jonathan Swift's 1726 satirical novel *Gulliver's Travels*, the protagonist visited the nation of Luggnagg, somewhere near Japan. Occasionally, a baby would be born with a red dot above their left eyebrow. These babies were called Struldbruggs. The red dot was a sign that they would never die. At first, Gulliver thought that this long life would be a monumental gift leading to great wisdom and wealth, but later he realized that these poor creatures aged normally, acquiring progressive tragic disability along the way, without the gift of death to end their suffering. Swift was powerfully illustrating the reality that survival alone is not a proper goal for aging, a truth he would come to know before dying with dementia at the age of 78.[II,3]

The term "homeostasis" refers to all of the processes responsible for managing and adjusting the activities of the body to maintain stability and resistance to challenges. It is necessary to consider homeostasis beyond the concept of disease avoidance, as there is more to health than the absence of disease. This is illustrated by the word "salutogenesis," which describes the promotion and maintenance of health.[4] This is in contrast to pathogenesis, which is the promotion and maintenance of disease. Salutogenesis illuminates the vital concept that health is not a passive process and that we can make a difference in taking control of factors that determine our health and fitness. Likewise, the concept of considering "healthspan" as opposed to "lifespan" demonstrates that the goal should be obtaining years of active meaningful survival, not just survival itself.[5]

Salutogenesis illuminates the vital concept that health is not a passive process and that we can make a difference in taking control of factors that determine our health and fitness.

[II] A discussion of Swift's memory disorder is presented in reference 3.

Because the body systems that have reduced function with age are all dependent on each other, declines in function can have magnified effects throughout the body. Interactions between our body systems not only affect our susceptibility to disease, but also our functional capacity with aging. Recognition of this interdependence is a critical factor for successful aging and is the focus of this book.

Aging Is Not Inevitable

As we will see later, the ability of older people to survive illness and maintain fitness is determined not only by the illness itself, but also upon the reserve factors of the person to adapt (as discussed in Chapter 2). It is our reserve factors which maintain the balance of body functions, even in the presence of challenges, such as disease and other sources of stress. Our reserve capacity is another way to present the concept of resistance to loss of function. The maintenance of health and fitness is an active process, which is dependent in large part upon our activities, attention, and attitude.

The importance of our attitude in regard to aging – and where that attitude is often misdirected – is illustrated by the popular phrase "aging is inevitable." It isn't. Yet the myth is widespread. A recent review of aging and the cardiovascular system (2020) noted that "Aging is an inevitable part of life."[6] I disagree, as many people do not live long enough to get to be old. Aging is not inevitable, because it doesn't happen to everyone.

Aging is not inevitable, because it doesn't happen to everyone.

What would Princess Diana, John F. Kennedy, or Martin Luther King Jr. think about the idea that aging is inevitable, as Diana died at the age of 36, John F. Kennedy at 47, and Martin Luther King Jr. at the age of 39? We all know people who did not live long enough to be old, so we must conclude that aging is not inevitable. On the other hand, aging is an opportunity. To put it another way, everyone is certainly one day older today than they were yesterday, but not everyone will be one day older tomorrow than they are today because our survival from one day to the next is not guaranteed.

One reason that aging is not inevitable is that many people do not reach the ages at which they are considered to be "old" (usually 65 years of age in Western cultures). Of all persons born 65 years ago in the United States, only 86 percent are still living. In the same vein, a 65-year-old person should not assume that they will live to be 80 because of the idea that aging is inevitable. At the time of writing, according to the United States Social Security Administration, a healthy 65-year-old man has a 62 percent probability and a healthy 65-year-old woman a 71 percent probability of living to be 80 years old (see www.ssa.gov/OACT/TR/2021/index.html).

Second, and most importantly, aging is not inevitable because the declines of function seen with aging can often be avoided. Yes, that's the reality of aging.

For example, a 60-year-old woman with coronary artery disease could improve her cardiac function with exercise, statins, improved diet, reduced alcohol intake, and quitting smoking, so that by the age of 70 her cardiac function would be better than it was at the age of 60. This does not imply that all age-related changes can be prevented, but many of the declines in function we see with aging are not produced by aging alone but are the result of harmful lifestyle behaviors that can be changed with significant effect.

What can be done to enhance the opportunity of aging?

Since many people do not get a chance to be old we should not consider our survival to be inevitable. We should reflect on what can be done to enhance the opportunity of aging. To this end, we should all be asking ourselves two central questions:

> How can we influence the quality and length of our lives through lifestyle measures, in consideration of the interdependent forces we have been discussing?
> How can we maximize the meaning of our lives to make the most of the opportunity presented by aging?[7]

Many people, including some medical professionals, have a shockingly negative view of aging. Consider a 2020 report published in *Lancet* entitled "Ageing without dementia: can stimulating psychosocial and lifestyle experiences make a difference?"[8] Written by leaders in the field of gerontology, its authors argue that "ageing is the accumulation of biological deficits resulting from genetically and environmentally induced alterations that undermine the homeostatic balance of the organism, progressively leading to physical and cognitive impairment."[8]

Let's take a moment to unpack this. In aging, there are deficits in bodily functions related to genes and environment. These declines interfere with the ability of the body to maintain health and fitness. So far, so good. The problem is in the last phrase when the authors suggest "physical and cognitive impairment" is inevitable. *It is not.*

As you will see in the following chapters, many older people do not suffer cognitive losses, and people, as they age, may build muscle mass and improve abilities as they get older through physical exercise. A remarkable feature of aging is that even in later stages of life there are recovery mechanisms which help to retain function in the face of structural decline.

Although it is true that there are declines with aging, they do not always cause physical and cognitive impairment.

For example, a 50-year-old runner may be able to increase their performance over the 10 years until the age of 60 through improved training. Although it is best for people to learn to play a musical instrument in childhood, it can be done in adulthood. An enthusiast who starts violin lessons at the age of 50 will not be playing with the New York Philharmonic. But she can, through teaching and practice, obtain sufficient skill to develop the potential for decades of joy from music making. Many older people work hard throughout their life and find that their later ages are the most joyful of all.

In order to consider what can be done to improve our aging we must first consider how we are affected by aging.

What Is Happening with Aging?

Now that we understand the three goals, and the concept that aging is not inevitable, we must consider the reality of human aging. What is happening?

Aging is accompanied by the reduced function of every system of the body (see Figure 1 and Table 1). What's important to know is that this reduced function is not a disease, it's highly variable from person to person, and does not necessarily lead to impairment in activities. Although every organ has reduced function with aging, this decline is accompanied by increased variability.[10] This means, as shown in Figure 2, that walking speed typically declines with age. But that's not true for everyone. While most young people walk at similar rates, some older people walk as fast as younger people, while others slow dramatically. Many older persons will maintain function in later life. This is not the case only for walking speed, as the variability of every measure of body structure and function is greater for older than for younger persons. This is powerful evidence that aging declines do not happen to everyone and that it matters what we do about the opportunity for aging.

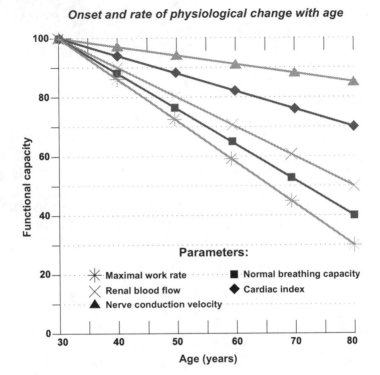

Figure 1 Declines in function with aging
All bodily functions decline with age. This includes maximal
work rate, blood flow in the kidney, maximum breathing
capacity, nerve conduction velocity, and cardiac output, as well
as many other functions. The lines indicate the relative declines
in function from ages 20–30 to 80–85. These changes do not
represent a disease and do not occur to the same degree in every
person. (Adapted with permission from reference 9.)

An important thing to realize about reduced function in aging is that in many cases normal function can
be maintained through healthy lifestyle choices. For example, 30–50 percent of centenarians (aged 100 years or
older) are cognitively intact. Muscle mass declines with
age, but some people have excellent muscle mass even

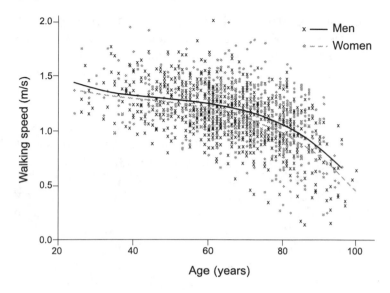

Figure 2 Variability increases with age
Usual walking speed declines with age, particularly after the age of 65. However, there are many people over 65 years old who have a normal walking speed. The data for the younger ages are more closely aligned to the average, while older persons have considerably more variation in their walking speed. This increase in variability with aging is true for every aspect of function. (Adapted with permission from reference 11.)

after 65 years, and it's possible for most people to build muscle mass through exercise, no matter the age. Some of the declines with aging noted in studies of older people are not caused by aging alone, but by the early stages of disease that may be present in a premature state which is difficult to detect (such as Alzheimer's disease).[12]

This is what happens in the brain with aging: There is a reduction in brain volume, which is more marked in areas involved in learning and memory. The structure of the myelin sheath, which isolates axons connecting neurons, also declines. This activates the immune system in the brain, which needs to repair the damage. Abnormal collections of proteins develop in the brain along with impaired removal of toxic molecules, and loss of synapses (gaps between nerve cells responsible for communication). There is also improper folding of brain proteins with aging. (This is a critical concept in aging and is discussed in Chapter 5.) Inflammation in the brain produces molecules which impair learning. All of these age-related changes in the brain can lead to a loss of function as we grow older. Cognitive activities at work and at home can help delay these changes and enhance our cognitive reserve; such activities are closely related to psychological factors and social interactions. Furthermore, it has been discovered recently that important immune cells in the brain which are involved in learning and memory are strongly influenced by gut bacteria (our microbiota). And these organisms are controlled by what we feed them (our diet!). So, our microbiota are a key component of our physical reserve.

We need to consider what happens to our immune system with aging, because it is central to the preservation of function as we get older. Also, we are able to influence the nature of our immune system through our actions, as we shall soon see.

The Immune System in Aging

The immune system is an intricate network of cells and molecules, which protects us from infections and assists in the maintenance of structure. It plays a vital role in aging in the body as well as in the brain. Inflammation is a protective mechanism which allows us to fight infection and defends us from disease-causing agents. *Innate immunity* refers to the system providing initial rapid defenses, independent of previous exposures, with no memory (repeat exposures are treated the same) and lasting only a few days (such as the body's initial response to a cold).

Adaptive immunity is slower to develop, involves immune cells, and lasts a lifetime (such as vaccinations). There may be activation of the innate immune system with aging, which is found in many neurological and systemic disorders and has been called "inflammaging."[2] Difficulties can develop when inflammation is ineffective and pathogens enter, replicate, and damage tissues. However, it is also a problem when inflammation is excessive. Immune mechanisms can be active (pro-inflammatory) or regulatory (anti-inflammatory).

With aging, there are often excessive pro-inflammatory factors and inadequate regulatory mechanisms. This low-grade process of inflammaging is linked to several diseases of aging, such as cardiovascular disease, stroke, diabetes, Alzheimer's disease, Parkinson's disease, and cancer.[2] Chronic low-grade inflammation can cause cellular damage in localized areas of the body and also influence cellular process at remote sites. In addition, the production of growth factors in the brain may be impaired by inflammation, and inflammatory molecules may damage neurons, increase the production of misfolded proteins involved in many age-related brain diseases, and increase the assembly of free radicals. Free radicals are highly reactive molecules with unpaired electrons produced by metabolism, which damage other things, such as carbohydrates, DNA, and proteins and impair cellular structures, such as the mitochondria, which is the source of the cell's energy.

The inflammation in the brain is linked to the inflammation in the body. The wonderful part of this is that the bacteria in the gut strongly influence these processes, both in the brain and the body. Excessive inflammation in the body and brain can be caused by a diet which enhances the growth of gut bacteria that enhance inflammation. And inflammation can be reduced with the presence of health-enhancing bacteria, also related to diet.

This means that our diet can contribute to an unhealthy pro-inflammatory state or a health-enhancing regulatory, anti-inflammatory state.

The brain is protected from the circulation by the blood–brain barrier, which tightly regulates the entry and exit of molecules and cells from the blood to the brain and vice versa. Despite the actions of the barrier the brain hosts an important population of immune cells that have been present from birth and also cells that regularly cross the barrier and monitor the health of the brain. Recent research has shown that these cells are needed for learning and memory as well as protection from pathogens.

As neurons age they release factors that increase inflammation in the brain, which through the activity of immune cells and related molecules can be damaging. It is a delicate balance of function that controls these processes, which are influenced by genetic and environmental factors, including diet and the microbiota (all the microbes that reside inside our body and on our surfaces). If the inflammatory process becomes excessive it can lead to neurodegeneration.[13] Inflammation can also affect the brain directly, such as with meningitis, encephalitis, or brain abscess. Dormant microbes in the brain that are not replicating can also influence inflammation without active infection. The DNA of microbes can become implanted in human DNA sequences and influence metabolism, even without replication of the microbe. Inflammation elsewhere in the body can also affect the brain through the passage into the brain of inflammatory cells and molecules.

The balance of inflammation in the brain can often become poorly regulated with aging. This can result from poor clearance of toxic molecules from the brain, increased production of inflammatory molecules, abnormally folded proteins, fewer neuroprotective factors (growth factors), and changes in the gut microbes. These factors can act in a dangerous feed-forward loop in which inflammation leads to more protein misfolding, leading to more inflammation. These processes which impact inflammation and protein folding are linked to our activities through life, including toxic exposures (such as smoking, alcohol, toxins, and chemicals), poor diet, head injury, and a lack of physical and mental activity. This means that it is possible to reduce our risk of poorly regulated inflammation as we get older by making proper lifestyle choices. Although the ability of the brain to deal with improperly folded proteins decreases with age it is possible to enhance our capacity to manage errors in protein folding. Dietary factors as well as mental and physical activities (presented in Chapter 20) can help manage the processes of inflammation.

The management of changes in inflammation with aging are important for the maintenance of function and avoidance of disease in everyone. Why are these issues especially important for older persons?

Old Persons Are Not Well Protected by Evolution

Evolution has not prepared us for a long life. Human evolution is critical to understanding human aging, so let's briefly explore it. It is estimated that our species, *Homo sapiens*, is one of the youngest of all life forms on Earth. We may only be about 100,000 years old as a species. At first glance, that number may seem high, but in comparison, chimpanzees – our closest relatives – are five to seven *million* years old. So, chimps have been here about 60 times longer than us. For almost all of human history, we have been living as hunter–gatherers with a profoundly different lifestyle than the one that we have today. Hunter–gatherers are nomadic people who live by harvesting wild food through hunting and fishing. The genes we have inherited were chosen by natural selection because they aided the survival of our ancestors, who were living in a different world than the one we are living in today. To be blunt, our genes do not prepare us for modern life, or, as you will see, old age.

For most of human history (perhaps prehistory would be more accurate), there were few people who grew old, because of infectious diseases, injuries, and scarce resources. Only a small percentage of the population lived to be over 65 years of age. From 1990 to 2020, the percentage of Americans aged 65 years and older has gone from about 4 percent of the population to nearly 20 percent of the population. Currently, about 9 percent of the world's population is 65 years of age or older. For most of human history, the percentage of the population who lived to be 65 years of age or older was just 3 percent. Studies of the teeth of ancient communities show that few persons lived long lives. In fact, life expectancy for most of human history was about 25 years. This is all to say that our genetic inheritance does not prepare us well for old age.

This is all to say that our genetic inheritance does not prepare us well for old age.

In short, evolution doesn't care about our survival to old age. What is essential to evolution is the dissemination of genes to the next generation. As far as evolution is concerned, it is imperative that we live long enough to have and raise children so our genes can be passed on. Survival into old age does not influence the passage of our genes.

This is not an ethical or a moral issue, it is just the way evolution works through natural selection. Thus, genes which decrease the chance of living to be 20 years of age will be diminished in the population by negative selection, because people with the genes linked to early death will raise fewer children. On the other hand, genes which make it likely that one will not live to be 70 years old after they have survived to 40 years will not be subject to such negative selection because few people have children over the age of 40 years. To put it in another way, genes which enhance survival to 70 years of age after reaching 40 years will not be selected for, because they will not enhance the occurrence and survival of offspring. Of course, genes that enhance survival in early life may very well continue to enhance survival in later years. But genes with a small positive effect in early life, but a negative effect in later life, will be favored by evolution, because there are so many more children than older persons.

Scientists have debated whether grandparents aid the survival of their grandchildren because of their wisdom and knowledge of the world.[14] Grandmothers, in particular, are thought to have enhanced transmission of cultural knowledge and complex social connections. While this is certainly true, it must be balanced by the fact that, until recently, older and possibly disabled older persons compete for scarce resources, which may decrease the survival of their offspring.

Let's consider aging in the context of the past 100,000 years of human history, since that is the time when our genes were selected. Our ancestors did not have access to plumbing, electricity, books, grocery stores, hospitals, doctors, or cell phones (and agriculture is only about 10,000 years old). As we touched on above, our genes were selected because they were adaptive to us in the environment in which we were living around 100,000 years ago, not because they are adaptive in our current environment. For example, the most important nutritional problem our distant ancestors experienced was not having enough to eat. The foods available to our ancestors were not as high in calories as foods that are readily available today – they ate more vegetables, less meat, and no processed foods. In contrast, the most important nutritional problem today in middle- and high-income countries is having too much to eat. We have not had this situation of nutritional excess long enough to develop effective genetic mechanisms to protect ourselves from overeating. Similarly, our ancestors were physically active out of necessity. If not, they would have had little to eat or drink and, perhaps, die. Even today, many people around the world need to travel every day to get water.

So evolution favors youth. The situation is different for older people – we are not really made to live that much longer than 40 or 50 years. People over 50 years of age are not as well protected from disease and loss of function. This doesn't mean that aging itself is a disease, just that the balance of health is more delicate with advancing age. One way to consider this is to imagine a group of 70-year-old men playing American-style football. There would be a stretcher on the field after every play and a long line-up of ambulances would be required.

The bottom line here is that survival to late years of age has been a relatively uncommon event in the 100,000 years of human history. Very few people got to be old until the twentieth century. Older persons are not as well prepared to face the stresses of the world because of the evolutionary factors discussed above. *As a result, it is necessary for older persons to consider the effects of their lifestyle choices on their four reserve factors and their ability to age successfully.* Awareness of these factors is important for our appreciation of the impact which our activities have on our aging.

Our ancestors were more physically active than many people are today. Were they also more mentally active? Years ago, I was backpacking with my son in a side ravine of the Grand Canyon in Utah. Even though we had a guide, we got lost and found ourselves deep in a canyon, and two miles away from our campsite when the sun set. It was dark and we had no flashlights (and cell phones with lights were 20 years away). After an hour of uncomfortable scrambling, we were relieved to see a full moon appear directly above us, lighting the path back to the campsite and helping us avoid stepping on rattlesnakes. As we walked, a thought occurred to me. Would the moon travel on a path parallel to the canyon, allowing for a few hours of moonlight, or would the moon travel on a path perpendicular to the canyon, in which case its light would soon be gone? I realized that this was the first time in my life that I had considered the path the moon was taking in the sky. In contrast, 20,000 years ago, our ancestor's awareness of the cycles of the moon were vitally important for their survival.

It is likely our ancestors were more mentally active than many people are today. To live in intimate daily contact with the natural world one needs to be continuously aware of the environment. In the absence of farming, refrigerators, and grocery stores, our ancestors needed to know where to find food, how to stalk, kill, and butcher animals, what was safe to eat and what was poisonous, and what time of year it could be found. Equally important was the danger of threats from neighbors, predators, insects, weather, and other hazards. People needed to be aware of the world for their own protection. Such a high level of awareness of the natural world is not required for survival today. For example, consider my highly reliable way to determine if a mushroom is safe to eat. I know one bite of certain mushrooms can fatally damage my liver. My method for mushroom safety evaluation is that I will not eat it if it is not wrapped in plastic, and not sold in a store. Learning mushroom identification was important for my ancestors but it's not one of my necessary skills.

These evolutionary considerations should frame our attention to the four reserve factors (cognitive, physical, psychological, and social). Because we are not "designed" by evolution for a long life, we must be prepared to use all the resources at our disposal to resist the challenges that we face as we get older. These reserve factors are needed to deal effectively with the many kinds of physical and mental stress that we all encounter. Resilience requires abundant resources in the brain, the body, and social ties as well as healthy ways of responding to life events.

Conclusion

The need for us to take an active role in our own aging is illustrated by an 1884 quote about the advance of democracy from the American poet James R. Lowell. "There is no good in arguing with the inevitable. The only argument available with an east wind is to put on your overcoat." Because aging is felt to be inevitable, people believe its manifestations cannot be altered. Understanding that aging is not inevitable allows us to prepare ourselves for a critical period in life's journey. Not only can we wear the metaphorical overcoat to protect ourselves from the forces of aging, we can also do things to affect the magnitude and characteristics of our own aging process.

I toyed with the idea of calling this book *Arguments with Aging*, to represent the need to be actively involved in the process of aging, and not passive observers. Staying healthy and active with a life full of meaning as we age requires fierce, tenacious attention to the factors that not only protect us from the winds of aging, but also change its forces and manifestations.

2 THE THEORY OF THE MULTIPLE RESERVE FACTORS

Education is what survives when what has been learned has been forgotten.

B. F. Skinner (1904–1990), American
behaviorist and psychologist

We have just reviewed how aging presents us with significant challenges to our survival, as well as to our function. The concept of the reserve factors allows us to appreciate the resources that we need to meet these challenges. As we age, our bodies need these reserve factors to rush into action and help us respond well to the stresses of our lives.

I propose that our four reserve factors serve to maintain our function and allow us to withstand the declines of aging and the demands of life events:

1. **Cognitive reserve** is made up of the brain's ability to work effectively, perform its higher functions, and maintain resilience despite challenges.
2. **Physical reserve** is the capacity of all the body's systems (cardiovascular, pulmonary, musculoskeletal, gastrointestinal, microbiota, and others) to perform well despite the changes caused by aging and the challenges that develop.
3. **Psychological reserve** is our ability to maintain healthy mental function and avoid agitation, anxiety, depression, and other unhealthy mental states.
4. **Social reserve** describes our interpersonal networks and support systems and our ability to be connected to others and society.

The concept of the reserve factors is illustrated by this scenario. Imagine if Roger Federer was made to carry a 50-pound pack on his back during a tennis match. Surely, his function would decline, but not as much as weekend athletes. I am a so-so amateur tennis player. If I were forced to carry a 50-pound pack on my back, my abilities would be more severely impaired than those of Roger Federer because I have a much lower reserve capacity compared to the man who has won multiple Australian Open, Wimbledon, and US Open titles. This is because I'm a less talented tennis player (you should see my backhand) and have less physical capacity than Federer. In short, I have a lower level of physical reserve than he does.

All four reserve factors contribute directly to protection from the Alzheimer's disease process in the brain, as well as influencing the changes in cognitive function with aging. All of these factors contribute to the ability of a person to maintain function in the face of trials which may impair cognition. We will start the discussion of the four reserve factors with a review of cognitive reserve.

Cognitive Reserve Factor

The fitter our brain is, the more it can withstand impairment from aging or disease.

The fitter our brain is, the more it can withstand impairment from aging or disease. In the 1980s, a mentor of mine, Robert Katzman, together with other colleagues at the Albert Einstein College of Medicine in New York, showed that education was protective against the development of Alzheimer's disease. People who were more educated had a lower risk of getting the disease and had onset at later ages than people with less education. The advantage provided by education was originally referred to as

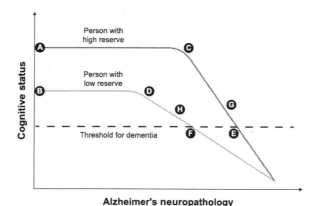

Figure 3 Cognitive reserve factor
People with more cognitive reserve start at a higher level
of cognitive function (A) than persons with low cognitive
reserve (B). Because of this, people with high cognitive reserve
will show declines later in life (C) and develop dementia later
(E) than persons with low reserve (D, F). Persons with a high
level of cognitive reserve may show more rapid decline after
onset of impairment (G) than persons with low reserve (H).
(Adapted from reference 15.)

"neuronal reserve." In more recent times it is known as
cognitive reserve, which has also been referred to as cerebral reserve, brain reserve, cognitive flexibility, or resilience (see Figure 3).[15]

One meta-analysis[16] showed a 7 percent decline in the
risk of dementia with each additional year of education.[I]
In our studies in Israel, in an Arab community, we found
that even a few years of education have a protective effect.

Education is not the only measure of cognitive activity,
of course. Many people who are denied education don't go
on to have stimulating occupations because of economic
or other social factors. However, those same people may

[I]   A meta-analysis is a systematic summary of previously obtained
research data.

write poetry, or enjoy solving differential equations. A person's mental life cannot be defined by their education or occupation. My research group published the results of a study in 2001, showing that a higher cognitive demand of occupational activities is associated with a lower risk of dementia with aging. The study focused on the effect of non-occupational activities in middle-aged people, both at work and at home, in midlife (ages 20–60).[17] My reasons for choosing this focus was that I felt educational and occupational activities were not a complete measure of a person's mental activities.

Our study of non-occupational activities included 193 people with Alzheimer's disease and 358 people without the disease. The chance of being in the Alzheimer's disease group was nearly four times higher for people who had less than the average number of activities. People with Alzheimer's disease were more likely to have participated in fewer intellectual activities. Several studies by others support the conclusion that cognitive activities either in school, at home, or at work reduce the risk of dementia.[17,18]

Do Alzheimer-Related Changes in the Brain Always Cause Impairment?

About one-third of people over the age of 65 years who have neuroimaging or neuropathological evidence of Alzheimer's disease do not have dementia. These individuals may have been protected by high levels of the cognitive reserve factor. Studies of centenarians in the Netherlands show that subjects with both amyloid plaques and neurofibrillary tangles in the brain often remain cognitively normal for years despite Alzheimer-related changes in the brain. This led the authors to conclude: "Dementia is not inevitable at extreme ages, which may be explained by resilience against Alzheimer's hallmarks and risk factors."[19]

Physical and mental activity enhances the production of new neurons in the brain and increases the secretion of growth factors that help delay the progression of Alzheimer's disease. This is surprising and encouraging. In other words, a person's behavior is determined not only by the progress of the of disease but also the ability of the brain to deal with the disease.

Physical and mental activity enhances the production of new neurons in the brain and increases the secretion of growth factors that help delay the progression of Alzheimer's disease.

What Time Periods Are Important for the Development of Alzheimer's Disease?

Before the onset of memory loss, there is a long presymptomatic period during which the Alzheimer's disease process develops in the brain. As we will see in the chapter on neurodegenerative disorders (Chapter 5), the pathological process in Alzheimer's disease begins two decades or more before the initial symptoms are observed: it is a slow process allowing a long period during which interactions among brain pathways – including psychological, social, and environmental factors – may develop. The brain changes in the age-related neurodegenerations develop over many years, and the impaired function which is the outcome of these changes is not apparent until the structural loss in the brain becomes substantial.

The Nun Study of Aging and Alzheimer's Disease was an innovative, long-term study that illuminated many aspects of aging. Begun in 1986, it examined the lives of 678 Roman Catholic nuns in America. The study included psychological tests and post-mortem examinations. Investigators found that early-life linguistic ability was related to late-life cognitive decline and Alzheimer's disease neuropathology. It is also believed that they were protected by their high level of social interactions throughout their lives.[20,21] The researchers also found that many sisters had brain pathology suggestive of Alzheimer's disease but they remained cognitively intact until death, many in their 80s and 90s.

The relationships between cognitive activities and cognition are important in all stages of life. Cognitive activities in the early, middle, and later years are all protective against cognitive decline.[8] David Bennett and colleagues in Chicago have shown[22] that "early life cognitive enrichment" (intellectual stimulation) is associated with reduced Alzheimer's disease pathology later in life as well as less cognitive decline.[II] The influence of mental activities may delay the onset of dementing illness through the enhancement of cognitive reserve. Because the onset age of Alzheimer's disease is so late in life (usually after age 70) a delay of only a few years can have a big impact.

This is good news for all of us. Things that we do over the many decades of midlife and late life can influence these brain changes with aging because they develop so slowly. As we will see in Chapter 15, we can enhance our cognitive reserve factor through participation in mentally stimulating actions throughout our lives.

What Does Learning Do to the Structure of the Brain?
Mental activities, including memory, reading, speaking, perception, understanding, abstraction, music, and art (and many other functions of the brain) all involve the activation of neurons and neuronal networks (complex

---

[II] Considerable excellent work on cognitive reserve has also been done by Yaakov Stern and his group at Columbia University in New York City.

patterns of interconnected neurons). These processes all cause elevated cerebral metabolism of glucose and oxygen, increased cerebral blood flow, and the production of neuronal elements involved in cell-to-cell communication (dendrites and axons). This means that the structure of the brain is changed by learning.

Learning sparks brain activity, which has healthy benefits.

Learning sparks brain activity, which has healthy benefits. When you read a non-fiction book and begin to see connections to new things, your brain is stimulated. When you use a mobile phone language app on your phone, your brain is stimulated. Complex social interactions as part of a volunteer activity may also stimulate your brain. These actions create tiny, yet important, changes on a molecular level, known as "neuronal activity" or the electrical firing of neurons.

Neuronal activity also increases the production of new neurons and growth factors, as well as more cerebral capillaries – further boosting cognitive reserves. All mental processes involve the electrical activity of neurons (neuronal firing) and this neuronal firing inhibits neuronal degeneration. Neuronal activity is central to the health of the brain. It promotes the production of neurotransmitters, resistance to over-excitation, protection from toxins and free radicals, repair of DNA damage, enhanced intricacy of the tree of neuronal connections (neuronal networks), improved regulation of the stress response, and better and more healthful processing of disease-related proteins. Mental activities also keep the brain flexible. This is of particular value with aging, as alternate strategies can mask the presence of functional decline.

A recent study shows[23] that neuronal activity also enhances the function of the cells lining cerebral blood vessels, improving the function of the blood–brain barrier.[III] The blood–brain barrier is like a fence with serious security features that controls entry and exit to regulate the brain's environment to keep it healthy.

The benefits of this neuronal activity apply, as well, to other forms of dementia. Higher levels of cognitive reserve will be protective against the impairment in mental status caused by other illnesses, such as Pick's disease, Lewy body disease, and Parkinson's dementia as well as vascular cognitive impairment.

Physical Reserve Factor

Cognitive function is an accomplishment of the brain, and our level of cognitive function is dependent upon many factors including neuronal activity, metabolism, cerebral blood flow, and cognitive reserve capacity. But this is not enough. The brain's abilities to perform is dependent on several non-neurological matters, including interactions with all of the body's systems and the microbiota. Impaired function of the heart, kidneys, lungs, hematological, and other systems can affect brain function. Actions of the immune system are also a critical component of physical reserve.

The physical reserve (sometimes called systemic reserve) factor includes many elements of the body: the function of the brain and peripheral vessels, hypertension, diabetes, kidney, heart and pulmonary function, polypharmacy, sensory deficits, inflammation, nutrition, and the microbiota. The microbiota contribute to this reserve factor by helping preserve cognitive function. As discussed in Chapter 21 on

---

[III] The blood–brain barrier is a critical component of the brain's circulation. It protects the brain from entry of potentially harmful agents from the blood, controls exit of molecules from the brain, and is essential for maintenance of a healthy brain.

the microbiota, the complexities of the gut influence inflammation, and can be responsible for over- or underactive immune responses in the body.

When you exercise, something called brain-derived neurotrophic factor (BDNF) is generated. BDNF is a growth factor for neurons which enhances memory and learning. This is a lovely protective effect of riding your bike, running, shooting hoops, or participating in a sweaty class at the gymnasium. You cannot buy BDNF in the store and, if you could get it, it would have to be injected directly into the spinal fluid. But you can get more of it from exercise! It is well established that physical exercise increases the health of blood vessels (lower blood pressure) and aids cognitive function in later ages.[8] Exercise helps keep your blood pressure lower. A healthy lifestyle in early life, such as a good diet and physical activity, improves cognition in later life.

A healthy lifestyle in early life, such as a good diet and physical activity, improves cognition in later life.

The complexity of the physical reserve factor is best illustrated by smoking. Data suggest that cigarette smoking is a risk factor for Alzheimer's disease. This may be because of the toxic effect of the addiction on the brain and the brain's circulation. Smoking impairs circulation throughout the body, particularly in the heart and kidneys, and also causes impaired respiratory function. A lifetime of smoking damages cardiac, respiratory, circulatory, immune, and kidney function, in a way that reduces physical reserve and allows Alzheimer's disease to progress at a faster pace. Stopping smoking is an outstanding way of increasing physical reserve.

Chronic kidney disease is found in about 9 percent of populations worldwide. The kidneys manage our homeostasis and direct several functions, such as acid–base equilibrium, water balance, blood pressure control, and glucose levels. Brain function can easily be impaired by kidney problems in older persons.[24] Research has documented that the decline of kidney function in midlife is associated with a worse cognitive performance. Avoidance of diabetes and hypertension can help to preserve kidney function with aging. And the risk of diabetes and hypertension is related to diet, physical activity, and obesity.

Psychological Reserve Factor

Psychological reserve includes resilience from depression and stress, and effective responses to conflicts and grief. A high degree of psychological reserve involves the ability to use different strategies for coping with stress.[25] The early treatment of depression through behavioral or pharmacological means may help to delay the onset of Alzheimer's disease through increased participation in social tasks as well as physical and mental activities. Depression is a modifiable risk factor for Alzheimer's disease.[26] People who are emotionally more stable and have more resilience and conscientiousness have an increased resistance to cognitive impairment, even among those with markers of Alzheimer's disease in the brain.[27,28]

As people age, they often face a problem of diminishing gratification, as the rewards of work may be lost and, sadly, many persons have no interests outside of work. (It's really true: "All work and no play make Jack a dull boy." Pick up a hobby. Make friends. Join a group.)

The Austrian neuropsychiatrist Víktor Frankl has proposed that our search for meaning is a critical matter in our mental health. Meaning is often lost with aging because of the loss of work and the passing of friends and family members. Frankl said, "Those who have a 'why' to live, can bear with almost any 'how'." It is important that meaning be sought through life at all ages and that ways to preserve meaning with aging can be pursued. (See Chapter 16.)

It is important that meaning be sought through life at all ages and that ways to preserve meaning with aging can be pursued.

Withdrawal from the world limits the opportunity to integrate one's life in later years. It's important to stay involved in one's community through volunteering, talking, and listening to others, mentoring, making new friends, and finding joy in the world. According to psychoanalyst Erik Erickson, humans face a new challenge beginning at about the age of 65.[29] As people face the reality of a not-too-distant death, they must choose between integrity and despair. If a person feels a sense of accomplishment, acceptance, and some wisdom, then it is likely that they have landed at a healthy place of integrity. This is much better than the bitterness, regret, and hopelessness one has when surrounded by feelings of despair. Finding integrity isn't easy because aging may be accompanied by losses which damage our reserve capacity. Clearly, it is in our interest to strengthen our reserve factors in early life.

With aging, there is often a shift from doing to thinking, from planning to reminiscing, and from preoccupation with everyday events and long-range planning to reviewing and rethinking one's life. This may be a problem for people with early life trauma, who might have spent most of their time fighting off their memories. As cognitive function declines, they may have difficulty stopping harmful memories from returning. These interactions can lead to depression, social isolation, and a reduced capacity of the reserve factors to protect them from cognitive losses.

The concept of the psychological reserve factor helps to clarify the need to recognize the importance of mental health with aging. We must not wait for challenges to prepare our response mechanisms. We should enhance our psychological reserves by learning to practice acceptance, finding meaning and being actively engaged with others and the world.

Social Reserve Factor

Social reserve is comprised of family resources and other social networks, including marriage, occupational and recreational activities, money, environmental stimulation, and engagement or isolation. The cognitive stimulation provided by social interactions is critical for health at all stages of life. For the past 100,000 years or more, our ancestors lived in community settings and the genes which we have now were adaptive to that environment. Our forebears had contact with multiple generations of their families. Excellent evidence shows that social support systems are critical for health. Socially stimulating activities improve cognition in elders, and better social networks means improved cognitive function with aging. Physical and cognitive inactivity is related to poverty, loneliness, and social isolation. This inactivity is also linked to dementia. Social isolation increases the risk of coronary artery disease and stroke. In experiments, disease model mice that lacked social, physical, and cognitive engagement suffered from Alzheimer's disease brain changes at higher rates than other mice.

Socially stimulating activities improve cognition in elders, and better social networks means improved cognitive function with aging.

Clearly, social bonds have desirable consequences at all stages of life. Resilient social support aids both health and longevity. Fitness and resilience are aided by strong social ties. Researchers from the University of California, Los Angeles, observed that people with Parkinson's disease who have fewer meaningful social interactions are at an increased risk for more severe symptoms. This may be related to impaired diet and exercise (see Case Study 1).

Friendships, close relationships with siblings, children, and lovers are extremely important to a healthy life. Who doesn't love being with people who make them laugh or people they can have a stimulating conversation with?

Lonely individuals may be twice as likely to develop Alzheimer's disease in late life than those who are not lonely, according to a study by researchers at the Rush Alzheimer's Disease Center in Chicago.[30] Loneliness is related to poor health and functional limitations, which cause impaired social participation and diminished contact with friends and relatives. Loneliness is also a risk factor for mortality. It has been noted that well-integrated people are more resilient when facing stress. Lonely people exercise less, eat less nutritious food, and are less likely to properly take prescribed medications. This is a major problem with aging because of the loss of family and friends with the passage of years.

One way to fight off loneliness is by developing strong social networks. Kentucky author Wendell Berry writes that community is "the smallest unit of health and that to speak of the health of an isolated individual is a contradiction in terms."[31] This is expressed poignantly by Quiz Kid Donnie Smith (as played by William H. Macy) in the movie *Magnolia* (1999). "I really do have love to give!" he said. "I just don't know where to put it!"

Loneliness is an especially important problem for women. In 1993, elderly men in the United States were nearly twice as likely as their female counterparts to be married and living with their spouse (75 percent versus 41 percent). Elderly women, on the other hand, were more than three times as likely than elderly men to be widowed (48 percent versus 14 percent). Thus, while most elderly men have a spouse for assistance, especially when health fails, most elderly women must face life's challenges alone.

It has been observed that people place greater emphasis on positive social connections as they get older, probably because of increased awareness of their mortality.[32] The development of positive social relationships in aging is a vital factor in determining happiness. People with an inappropriately negative view of aging may fail to make meaningful interactions because of their negative expectations. It is an important goal of this book to appreciate the opportunities provided by aging, because what we do makes a difference.

Case Study 1

An 82-year-old retired engineer brought in by his daughter is seen because of the rapid onset of marked memory failures. She noted that three months ago her father became forgetful, inattentive, and had trouble finding the right word. His daughter reported that he was unable to use a can opener, toaster, and other kitchen appliances. He also had trouble finding his way around, even in familiar surroundings. He had difficulty combing his hair, using the toilet, and was forgetful. By talking to the daughter, I learned that he was intact until three months ago when she visited him at home and found that he had not washed and was not eating. He no longer knew the details of his treasured stamp collection and did not know where he had put the key to his car. His wife of 45 years had died six months earlier, and it was believed that his function was good before that. I learned that his wife had never allowed him to do any work in the kitchen and that she had always been present in the car to tell him where to go. I ordered an MRI scan of his brain. The scan showed evidence of cortical atrophy, worse in the parietal lobes, suggestive of Alzheimer's disease. Blood tests and examinations did not reveal any other cause of cognitive impairment. It is likely that the relatively rapid progression of his illness was not related to a sudden onset or worsening of Alzheimer's disease pathology in the brain but rather a change in his social environment. After his wife died, his main support system was gone, and his cognitive deficits became clear.

This scenario is commonly encountered in older people who are doing well but have a loss of social support or acquire a systemic illness (also known as a "comorbidity"), and then develop a rapid onset of cognitive impairment. This often happens to people with urinary tract infections, coronary artery disease, pulmonary insufficiency, or medications. It can also be due to a change in social environment or onset of depression.

Conclusion

The four reserve factors discussed here are all related to each other; they are not distinct but are based on a complex network of interactions. Developing your cognitive, physical, psychological, and social reserves will lessen the effect of reduced brain function in later life. Furthermore, enhancement of these factors will also diminish the disease processes themselves. Evidence for these relationships is substantial (see Figure 4).

I refer to this reserve concept as "the theory of the multiple reserve factors." The word "theory" is used because

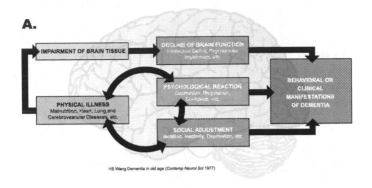

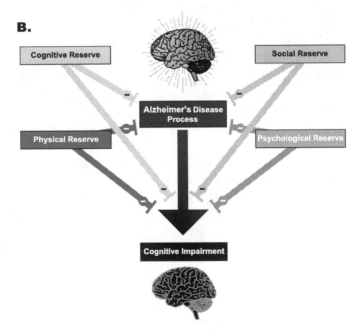

Figure 4 The four reserves and Alzheimer's disease
(A) This figure was produced by gerontologist H. S. Wang in 1977 to illustrate how the manifestations of dementia are the result of the interactions of cognitive, physical, psychological, and social factors. (Adapted with permission from reference 33.) (B) The four reserve factors all influence the development of the Alzheimer's disease process in the brain as well as the influence of that process on cognitive impairment. Each of the four reserve factors also interacts with all the others. The minus signs indicate that high levels of each of these factors serves to inhibit the Alzheimer's disease process in the brain as well as delay the development of cognitive impairment caused by the brain pathology.

the four reserve factors involve the most complex aspects of human life, over the course of a lifetime, and cannot be comprehensively evaluated with placebo-controlled, double-blind, randomized trials conducted over short time periods.[34] Despite this, there is already considerable evidence that supports the importance of these reserve factors.

Interactions and interdependencies have important implications for public policy. Government efforts aimed at enhancing the availability of education, increasing physical activities, and improving access to healthcare will reduce the severe personal and economic burden of neurodegenerative disorders associated with aging.

Consideration of the four reserve factors is essential for achieving the goals of aging. It is not enough to have good cognitive reserve if you cannot enjoy life because of physical impairments, social isolation, and an inability to appreciate the joy of living. It is not enough to have outstanding cardiovascular function if cognitive reserve has not developed in such a way that successful strategies and flexibility can maintain function. It is not enough to have excellent cognitive and physical reserve, but no interest in other people (poor psychological and social reserve). Life strategies can be developed to enhance the ability to develop and maintain all of these four reserve factors to augment the opportunities presented by aging.

The key word here is diversity. We must respect the needs of our diverse parts that allow us to meet our goals in aging. The concept of these four reserve factors is designed to frame our approach to lifestyle decisions, and an awareness of them is needed to enhance the goals of aging. Fortunately, there are many ways this can be accomplished, as we will see in Part II of the book, Chapters 12–25.

3 THE BRAIN IS NOT AN ORGAN, IT IS THE MASTER

The brain is a world consisting of a number of unexplored continents and great stretches of unknown territory.

Santiago Ramón y Cajal (1852–1934), Spanish neuroscientist, winner of the Nobel Prize in Physiology or Medicine, 1906

Is the Brain an Organ?

Before we consider the miracle of the brain, we must decide what to call it. We are taught through school and reading that the body has several organs. The second-century Greek physician Galen said that an organ is " … a part of an animal that is the cause of a complete action, as the eye is of vision, the tongue of speech, and the legs of walking; so too arteries, veins and nerves are both organs and part of animals." The word "organ" comes from the Greek *organon* for "instrument or tool," which is an object with a specific vital function.

The challenge in defining the brain's function is simple: the brain does not have just one function – it has all the functions.

Most of us know that the heart pumps blood throughout the body, the lungs absorb oxygen and discard carbon dioxide, and the kidneys filter the blood. But what exactly is the function of the brain? The challenge in defining the brain's function is simple: the brain does not have just one function – it has *all* the functions. Everything we do, whether consciously or automatically, is controlled or influenced by the brain. Aside from the obvious role of the brain in thought, consciousness, perception, attention, vision, hearing, taste, abstraction, anticipation, language, art, love making, and other processes, the brain is also busy monitoring everything that happens to us and managing the balance of our existence. The growth of hair is influenced by sex hormones produced by the gonads, under the influence of the pituitary glands that are coordinated by the brain. If we walk into a steakhouse and are confronted with the odor of grilled steak, our brain will send signals to the gastrointestinal tract to prepare for a high-fat meal. (And hopefully the brain will consider the impact of dietary decisions on health and choose a vegetarian or fish dinner, see Chapter 20.)

This list of roles that the brain plays in our lives could go on for a long time and is the subject of several books. (I recommend *The Idea of the Brain*[35].) Because of its many functions, I'd argue that it's not reasonable to consider the brain an organ. The problem with calling it an organ is that people have a tendency to lump it in with other organs, leading to an underappreciation of its profound complexity and importance. When we consider the brain to be an organ, we are framing our viewpoint in a restrictive way, enhancing the view that it is of an equivalent nature to other organs.

Awareness of the unique and central role of the brain in our lives helps us to appreciate the importance of its contributions. The brain is uniquely complex, adaptable, and sensitive to injury. When making decisions about what activities to pursue and what food to eat, always consider the welfare of the brain. It is a powerful and multifaceted essential part of the body.

My son's high-school biology textbook featured chapters on the organs of the human body. Each week, I'd ask him, "Are you studying the brain yet?" And each week he'd reply, "No." At the end of the semester, he told me his class never reached the chapter on the brain, because they didn't have enough time. You may be surprised to learn that a residency in internal medicine in the United States is three years in length, and during those 36 months, the internists in training study neurology for just one month. These are but two examples of the mistakes that develop when the brain is considered to be an organ.

Perhaps we could say, "The brain is not an organ, it is the organist." The musical instrument called the organ is the largest of all (and the only one requiring special shoes). Such an organ may have four different keyboards for the hands and one for the feet, and various controls for sound intensity and tone. It's a complex instrument, but the analogy stops there. With the organ, it's possible to see and appreciate the skill of an organist, and hear the result of the organist's work, but the brain's work is largely invisible.

I suggest that the brain be considered the hegemon: the master, commander, supreme leader, and chief.[1] I know that as a neurologist I am not an unbiased observer. But I feel that lack of respect for the brain and its role in our lives is a major problem. It is difficult for us to comprehend the brain as it is so very different from all other objects we have known, so it is hard to compare it to other things we have experienced.

Is the Brain a Computer?

The brain is the most complex object in the universe. Although it does computations, it is not a computer. The best way to see the difference is to consider a current-day

[1] I am is grateful to Shigehisa Kuriyama of Harvard University for suggesting that the brain is the organist, and Stavros Baloyannis of the University of Thessaloniki for suggesting that the brain is the hegemon.

laptop computer. If a computer scientist is given the laptop and asked what programs are uploaded on it, such a determination cannot be made if the computer cannot be turned on, and if no electrical or magnetic investigations can be conducted. The computer is physically static (not changing) in a material sense. Information is stored on the computer's hard drive, but this information is of an electromagnetic nature and is not maintained by anything a computer scientist can detect without devices. The brain, on the other hand, is not static, but dynamic (also called plastic). It is wonderfully adaptable.

The structure of the brain represents how it has been used and the structure of a computer represents only its potential use. The way a computer is used does not influence its structure, only its stored information. The brain is similar to a muscle, in that its structure and function are influenced by how it is used. But the complexity of this relationship is much more intricate for the brain, because it relates to all of our abilities, skills, talents, fears, hopes, and cognitive capacities – and let's not forget, consciousness. Unlike computers, the brain is not digital. Because of the brain's adaptability, our cognitive reserve is capable of change; it is intricately responsive to what we do. When we exercise vigorously, it increases our cognitive and physical reserve factors. Likewise, when we gorge ourselves on fatty foods, it decreases these reserves. This is definitely less of a problem for the young because they have plenty of both, but older people need to be much more thoughtful in their decisions about how much to exercise, what to eat, and nurturing healthy relationships in their lives.

Metaphor is a valuable mechanism for the representation of ideas, but all metaphors are approximations. When we say a person is a "shining star" we do not mean the person is a celestial body. Biologist Matthew Cobb has discussed the use of the metaphor of the brain as a computer,[35] and indicated that, by holding tightly to metaphors, we end up limiting what and how we can think: " ... we may indeed be approaching the end of the computational metaphor. What is not clear, however, is what would replace it." This is a central dilemma in understanding the brain. The brain is so monumentally complicated that there are no similar structures with equivalent complexity. So, we should be cautious in using metaphors to aid our understanding of the brain. Considering the brain to be a computer leads us to fail to appreciate its magnificent and vital adaptability and sensitivity.

Considering the brain to be a computer leads us to fail to appreciate its magnificent and vital adaptability and sensitivity.

The reason that the distinction between the brain and a computer is important is that it is vital to understand the capacity of the brain for change and the dependence of the brain upon the environment. (These attributes do not apply to computers.) Consider the little finger on the left hand of a cellist. The cellist's brain is very concerned and attentive to the position of this little finger, as its position determines the frequency of the sound produced by the string touched by that finger. When you hold a beer can, the relationship of the little finger to the other fingers of the left hand is of no concern – not so for the cellist. As cello students learn, they attend to the sounds produced by the different positions of the little finger, and therefore expand the connections between the receptors for position sense in their fingers and the brain regions involved in hearing. This plasticity of the brain is involved in all learning, as learning increases the complexity of neuronal connections, the density and size of neurons, the production of new neurons, the synthesis of neurotransmitter receptor proteins and growth factors, the density of blood vessels, the capacity for blood flow and metabolism, and even the resistance to toxic insults caused by free radicals or other products of metabolism. Recent studies suggest the formation of new synapses is managed by important cells in the brain which are not neurons but supporting cells called microglia, whose activities are modified by the body's microbes. This means that our capacity for learning is influenced by our gut microbes, illustrating an interaction of physical reserve (the microbiota) with our cognitive reserve (synapse formation). What we eat influences our gut bacteria, which affect our immune system, which influences the activities in the brain involved in learning. The practical impact of this important process is just beginning to be explored. This scenario is one of many reasons to choose a high-fiber diet low in saturated fat. And it provides further evidence that what we do makes a difference!

The Adaptability and Complexity of the Brain

We are capable of learning and memory because of the brain's profound adaptability and complexity. It is well known that the capacity of learning and the plasticity of the brain is greatest in early life, the best example being the ease of language learning in children. Kids growing up in bilingual households often learn two languages (or more) instead of just one. The brain's flexibility is also illustrated by the observation that in subjects blind since early life, an area of the brain involved in seeing, called the visual cortex, becomes involved in hearing, touch, and perception, as well as cognition.[36] A UK study measured the size of the brains of London cab drivers before and after learning the maze of the crazily complex streets in that city. In order to obtain a license to drive a cab, drivers must pass a rigorous exam on the streets of London known as "The Knowledge."

(I wish that such an exam was also required for taxi drivers in New York City.) Researchers discovered[37] that the size of the drivers' hippocampus, a brain region involved in recalling spatial relationships, grew after this arduous task.[II]

The remarkable adaptability and plasticity of a child's brain is not lost completely in older people, although it is reduced. Older people are certainly able to have new accomplishments. Consider Daniel Miller of Ohio, who played tennis in high school but stopped playing as he joined the US Navy to fight in World War II. He saw action during the D-Day invasion of Normandy. After the war he did not play again until the age of 50. He continued playing for the next 40 years with a remarkable record of achievement, winning both singles and doubles championships in his age group at US national tournaments. His final tournament win was in 2006 at the age of 90. Many times, he was ranked number one in his age group in the world. When I played him in 1997, he was 81 and I was 49. He was the number-one-ranked player in the world at the time. (I shouldn't hesitate to add that he was the number one player in the world amongst those of 80–85 years of age.) I narrowly defeated him, and I was exhausted at the end of the match; he was not. His outstanding physical reserve contributed to his survival to the age of 98.

There are few professional musicians who picked up an instrument after the age of 15, but it is possible for older adults to learn to play a musical instrument. Older people are able to learn new things, and there is no age at which significant learning is not possible. Claudio Monteverdi (1567–1643) wrote an opera at the age of 76, and Charles

---

[II]   The hippocampus is a brain region involved in memory, emotions, and spatial relations, which is shaped like a seahorse, hence the name hippocampus, the Latin name of the seahorse. The hippocampus helps us navigate life, not just space.

Darwin wrote an important book at the age of 72: *The Expression of Emotions in Man and Animals* (1872). Eric Kandel is a 91-year-old psychiatrist, winner of the Nobel Prize in Physiology or Medicine, who remains an active force in neuroscience. Claude Monet painted his great water lily landscapes in his 80s and Titian, Matisse, Picasso, and Michelangelo all remained creative in their 80s.

The complexity, sensitivity, and adaptability of the brain is key to understanding brain aging. While the work of muscle is contraction, and the work of the heart is pumping, the work of the brain is learning (along with everything else the brain does consciously or unconsciously). There are reportedly 86 billion neurons in the human brain. Each neuron may be connected to 10,000 or more other neurons. Neurons connect to one another with a small space between cells, called a synapse. Chemicals secreted into the synapse are called neurotransmitters. There are many neurotransmitters, communicating information from one nerve cell to another. Some of these are excitatory, which increase the firing rate, and some are inhibitory, which decrease the firing rate. Others are modulatory (they exert a controlling influence) and change the effect of other molecules. Some neurons use one neurotransmitter, and others may use several. There are also direct contacts between nerve cells which allow for communication without any chemical mediators.

Consider the complexity of the NASA space probe Juno, which has been orbiting the solar system's largest planet, Jupiter (five times farther from the Sun than Earth) since 2016. The spinning solar-powered ship is designed to help us understand the beginning of our solar system. Juno discovered that Jupiter's core is not solid and found water ice on its largest moon, Ganymede. Certainly, such an instrument as Juno is incredibly intricate and has complex wiring and advanced computers. Juno represents the height of human technological accomplishment. However, in terms of complexity, Juno is orders of magnitude simpler than the human brain.

We are greatly limited in our ability to understand the brain because of its complexity.

We are greatly limited in our ability to understand the brain because of its complexity. Of course, we would like to understand memory, perception, language, comprehension, and other advanced functions of the brain. And understanding how consciousness works presents an enormous challenge to scientists. As we consider problems of such great importance and difficulty, consider the fly. There are flies that can hover in flight and can change the angle of attack of their wings, in order to alter their position with incredible precision. We all know how hard it is to catch them! Even though they may have only about 130,000 neurons we cannot yet understand how they are able to maneuver in the air with such astonishing dexterity. It's not hard to see how we have not yet solved the problem of consciousness, if we have not yet comprehended how a fly can hover. Part of this problem is that brain research has been devoted largely to the study of neurons, and not behavior. British neuroscientist David Marr wrote:[38] "Trying to understand perception by understanding neurons is like trying to understand a bird's flight by studying only feathers. It just cannot be done."

It is widely believed that our understanding of the brain is fundamentally limited. As stated by cognitive scientist M. A. Minsky:[39] "If the brain was simple enough to be understood – we would be too simple to understand it!"

What we do know about the brain hints at its enormous complexity. Have you noticed that a movie camera placed on a walking filmmaker's shoulders produces a jerky recording, which is unpleasant to watch? But our head, which houses our eyes, is also connected to our shoulders. Why does our visual world appear so stable and calm for us, even when we move our head? The answer is that our inner ears contain a complex sensory apparatus which records with great precision the position of the head in space at every millisecond. This information is sent via nerves from the inner ear to the brain, and the brain calculates exactly what the eye muscles must do to balance the movement of the head so that our visual world is perfectly adjusted. This process involves the six muscles of each eye and also information about the position in space of the neck at every moment. And each eye muscle is controlled by a balance of excitation and inhibition. For example, when we look to the right, muscles on the right side of the eyes serve to pull the eyes over to the right. At the same time, the muscles on the left side of the eyes are relaxed to make it easier for the right-sided eye muscles to move the eyes. When the function of the nervous system is impaired, for example by alcohol, the activity of these intricate neuronal pathways is weakened and the result is the sensation of dizziness, difficulty walking, and falling.[III] This shows how the stability of our daily lives is an accomplishment of the brain achieved though complex networks of neurons.

Our experience of the "steadiness" of everyday life is a monumental achievement of the brain. The complex arrangement of receptors to detect position and movement, circuits of neurons (neural networks) to analyze the incoming information, and actions to maintain stability is beyond consciousness. We are not aware of these processes, but they are critical for our ability to act in the world.

[III] The inner ear structures involved in this process are the semicircular canals. In addition, the otolith organs in the inner ear perceive movements of the head in all possible directions, and tell us where the ground is at all times.

How Can We Understand the Brain?

The seventeenth-century anatomist Nicolaus Steno proposed that to comprehend the brain, we needed to take
it apart. This approach led to the study of brain function
from observing the effect of brain damage on behavior.
This line of inquiry has revealed many insights about the
localization of the function in the brain. Understanding
the fundamental processes such as consciousness has
proven to be more difficult to accomplish. This may be because "to locate the damage which destroys speech and to
locate speech are two different things," as observed by the
highly regarded nineteenth-century British neurologist,
John Hughlings Jackson.[40] To learn about the brain from
the study of the effects of damage is difficult when complex processes are studied. Disease in one part of the brain
will have a distant effect on other parts which are not actively involved in the illness.

Many neuroscientists say that in order to understand the
brain it is necessary to build one. This engineering focus
reveals a critical error in understanding. The human brain
is the product of evolution and not a product of a rational design process. The brain was not designed. Each step
in the evolution of the brain relied upon what had gone
on before. John Hughlings Jackson understood this and
pointed out how brain function is dependent upon evolutionarily older structures being dominated by newer ones.
That is, the development of our frontal cortices was not
the evolution of a new structure independently developed,
but rather an enhancement of what already existed. Jackson said that in evolution there is:[41] "... a gradual 'adding
on' of the more and more special, a continual adding on
of new organizations. But this 'adding on' is, at the same
time, a 'keeping down'. The higher nervous arrangements
evolved out of the lower keep down those lower, just as
a government evolved out of a nation controls as well as
directs that nation." No matter how hard we try to build a

brain, we will not end up with an organizational pattern the same as that of the brain itself.

The Vulnerability of the Brain

Case Study 2 provides a good example of the sensitivity of the aging brain to changes in the status of the body (physical reserve). This sensitivity is one of the most important features of the brain and is responsible both for its abilities (such as learning) as well as its vulnerability (to loss of function). Why is the brain so sensitive to change or to injury?

A child with a broken femur can recover completely, and the injured bone may be stronger after the injury than before. This result after damage cannot be said of the brain. Intact brain function relies not only on our neurons and supporting cells (called glia), but also on their connections. Even if neurons could be rebuilt after an injury, that may not be enough if their proper connections are not re-established. The brain is more sensitive to damage than any other structure in the body because of the incredible dependence of its structure on each person's unique development and environment. We can do well with half of our liver or with only one lung. But the brain is not capable of such incredible functional recovery after injury. Even though there are new neurons produced in the adult brain, they need to make the proper connections in order to allow for recovery. (The effects of head injury on the brain are discussed in Chapter 24.)

The brain is also sensitive to injury because of its high metabolic demands. It has about 2 percent of body weight and yet it utilizes about 20 percent of the oxygen and glucose we metabolize. This is because the electrical activity of neurons and their connections requires maintenance of ionic gradients across the nerve membrane. An ion is an atom or molecule with a net electric charge due to the loss

or gain of one or more electrons, and an ionic gradient occurs when there are more on one side of a membrane than
on another side. Every time a neuron is electrically active
with an action potential, the ions move across the cell membrane and the ionic gradient must then be re-established.
This process requires lots of energy, as neurons are active
throughout the day and night. Because of this the brain
must have a nearly constant supply of oxygen and glucose.

A rather old joke of mine may help to illustrate the sensitivity of the brain. Although it is widely believed that the
brain needs a constant supply of oxygen and glucose to retain function, it can be said that the brain can do perfectly
well without any supply of oxygen and glucose from the
blood for at least ... 30 seconds.

The cells in our bone marrow are constantly dividing
and replacing our blood cells (the average life of a red blood
cell is 115 days). Neurons are much less capable of replacement. This is understandable when you think again of the
cello student and the neurons responsible for the perception of the position sense in her left little finger. Her ability to play the cello is dependent upon the networks of
those neurons and the resulting control of the other parts
of her hand and arms, and the connections to the cortical
regions responsible for hearing and musical understanding. After injury, the replacement of those neurons may
not be helpful if they lack the proper connections that had
been established over decades of practice. The creation
and maintenance of these connections between neurons
is the structural basis of memory. They are also the foundation of our cognitive reserve.

---

*The creation and maintenance of these connec-
tions between neurons is the structural basis
of memory. They are also the foundation of our
cognitive reserve.*

Case Study 2

A clear example of interdependence between the brain and the rest of the body can be shown in a thought experiment. Imagine a healthy 80-year-old man who is doing well at home with no symptoms or signs of disease. His memory and cognition are working well, and he can drive safely, enjoy time with his grandchildren, and go for walks with his wife. Because of his age, it is expected that, compared to a 30-year-old, he has less cerebral blood flow, less glucose metabolism in the brain, decreased size and function of the neurons involved in memory and learning, some degree of shrinkage of the outer surfaces of the brain, less hemoglobin in the blood, fewer different bacterial species in the gut, reduced ability of his lungs to oxygenate his blood, reduced ability of his liver to metabolize toxins and produce needed serum proteins, and reduced function of his immune system to destroy invading viruses and other microbes that could cause sickness.

Now imagine that he develops a urinary tract infection, which is common in older men because of difficulty in the bladder emptying with an enlarged prostate gland. A 30-year-old man with such an infection may complain of pain upon urination and obtain a proper diagnosis and treatment with rapid resolution of the infection. Our 80-year-old subject may develop impaired memory and alertness, and possibly even have hallucinations and delusions. The key difference between the 80- and 30-year-old subjects may be that the several systems with declining function noted above contribute to more impaired brain function in the older person because of his reduced physical resilience, that is, less physical reserve. His liver's reduced ability to detoxify toxins may have not affected him before the infection, but now the bacterial toxins are more widely disseminated than in the case of the younger person and will impair brain function. His mild reduction in hemoglobin may have not been a problem before, but in the presence of the infection it may contribute to cerebral impairment. His immune response may have a reduced capacity to fight the infection and may also have an exaggerated production of immune molecules that create depressed cognitive function and delirium. A lack of diversity of his gut bacteria, often seen with aging, may contribute to an excess in activity of his immune system.

This incredibly common scenario serves to illustrate the complex interactions involving the brain and the rest of the body that occur in aging to determine health or disease. Moreover, it must be recognized that the outcome of such a scenario does not depend only upon the status of the brain, it also is dependent on the integrity of the various components of body function. With aging, we want to be free of heart diseases, such as congestive heart failure and others, of course. But that is not enough, as we also want to have as good heart and lung function as we can, in order to maintain resilience and the ability to resist the challenges to health and fitness which develop. We also wish to have healthy microbiota in the gut, to help provide a balanced immune response to challenges as well as assist in digestion and metabolism.

Making Memories and the Importance of Neuronal Connections

Making a memory involves creating a "memory trace" called an engram, the most basic unit of memory storage. The engram is central to the process of recording and storing experience. Imagine that you visit a friend who has acquired an extraordinarily beautiful cat. The neurons involved in that experience undergo persistent changes in their structure and function, which become the engram. Retrieval happens when this pattern of neuronal activation is repeated. Brain regions that may be involved in this engram include the visual cortex (what the cat looked like), the auditory cortex (the sound of its purring), the sensory cortex (what it felt like to touch), the temporal lobes (memory of other cats, longing for a cat you had previously known, words to describe the cat), as well as association cortical areas in the cerebral hemispheres that are involved in interactions of perceptions, language, memory, and other functions. The temporal lobes are involved in the task of producing, storing, and retrieving the engram. Also, the anticipation of what it might be like if the cat is angry and aggressive may stimulate fear and a plan for dealing with a potential attack. The frontal lobes will be involved in understanding the integration of these factors into behavior (e.g., "I don't know this cat, do I really want to touch this cat?"). And I'd rather not consider which regions are involved in contemplation of a more complex matter ("How will my cat react when I bring home a new baby?"), which cannot be localized. This scenario is presented to illustrate how all the cortical areas in the brain are involved in memory. Also, the nature of the connections between cortical areas gives each person their distinctive features.

The factors responsible for the uniqueness of each individual are primarily neurological. And this uniqueness is not only because of an abundance of certain populations of neurons, but rather the distinctiveness of their connections. To write poetry, for example, the poet must access brain networks involved in sensation, perception, semantics, memory, emotion, abstraction, language, imagination, and meaning. Also, these networks need to have the opportunity for interactions – it is critical that they are not extinguished through fear, anxiety, disturbed attention, pain, or depression.

The Brain and the Microbiota

It has recently been discovered that several aspects of brain functioning are influenced by bacteria and other microbes in the gut. Feeding a high-fat diet to pregnant mice alters brain development of the offspring, who may have features of autism spectrum disorder.[42,43] Relationships of gut bacteria to behavioral issues in children and older persons have now been well documented. The process of making connections from one neuron to another, which is critical to learning, is influenced by brain cells called microglia; these are the chief innate immune cells of the brain and "highly active guardians of brain homeostasis."[42,44] The microglia are the primary macrophage of the brain (cells that engulf and digest debris). Several hundred thousand synapses are in the territory of one microglial cell. These cells monitor the nervous system, scavenging the brain looking for hazardous agents, managing the consumption of dying neurons, and pruning non-functioning synapses as well as facilitating repair. The microglia also support neurons with growth factors and allow for establishment and destruction of synapses. They have been found to sculpt synapses, thus modulating learning and memory.[45] They also influence neuronal activity and have a role in epilepsy. Surprisingly, the microglia in the brain are strongly influenced by gut bacteria. The recently discovered relationship of the microbiota to microglia in the brain means that dietary intake influences learning and memory as well as the health of the nervous system. (We will learn about this in Chapter 8.)

The recently discovered relationship of the microbiota to microglia in the brain means that dietary intake influences learning and memory as well as the health of the nervous system.

The brain is dependent upon all of the body systems with which it interacts, including the microbiota. Adequate oxygen and glucose supply is required by the brain from its blood flow, as provided by systemic and brain blood vessels and the heart and lungs. Oxygen delivery is also dependent upon circulating red blood cells provided by the bone marrow and adequate pulmonary function. The brain must be free of toxic factors that can be present because of disorders of the liver and kidneys. The brain also requires adequate nutrition, which must be obtained from the gastrointestinal tract, including the liver. Changes in physical reserve may heavily impact cognitive reserve. These interactions are all critical at all stages of life, but especially sensitive in the later years of aging.

Conclusion

The goal of this discussion is to enhance our appreciation of the magnificent complexity of the brain. We must respect its central role in our lives and work to see what we must do to enhance its health throughout life.

The good news concerning the sensitivity of the brain is that there are many things we can all do to improve the health and fitness of the nervous system with aging. Our capacity to survive, avoid disease, and maintain health and fitness in later years is not dependent entirely upon our genes. Also, the brain is central to determining health in aging, but it does not operate alone. Cognitive reserve is heavily dependent on the other three reserve factors we've discussed: social, psychological, and physical. If we can pay attention to the opportunity provided by aging, we can use the magnificent plasticity of the brain and enhance our four reserve factors, thus increasing our resilience as we age.

4 MEMORY AND COGNITION

Memory: A Primary and Fundamental Faculty

At the age of 68, the American essayist, lecturer, and philosopher Ralph Waldo Emerson began having trouble remembering things. Sometimes he struggled trying to find the words he wanted to say or write. "Memory is a primary and fundamental faculty, without which none other can work; the cement, the bitumen, the matrix in which the other faculties are embedded; or it is the thread on which the beads of man are strung, making the personal identity which is necessary to moral action," he wrote in *The Natural History of the Intellect*.

"Without it all life and thought were an unrelated succession," Emerson continued. "As gravity holds matter from flying off into space, so memories give stability to knowledge; it is the cohesion which keeps things from falling into a lump, or flowing in waves ... Memory performs the impossible for man by the strength of his divine arms; holds together past and present, beholding both, existing in both, abides in the flowing, and gives continuity and dignity to human life. It holds us to our family, to our friends. Hereby a home is possible; hereby only a new fact has value."

It may be that Emerson's interest in memory was related to his developing cognitive difficulties. He later said, when asked how he was feeling, "Quite well; I have lost my mental faculties but am perfectly well." He died in 1882, after many years of progressive decline.

As expressed so well by Emerson, memory and cognition are critical parts of who we are. Our capacity for recall allows us to use past experience to guide present and future actions. The critical nature of memory obscures the vital roles of other cognitive functions. That is, it is easy to observe your own ability to remember things as well as the memory capacity of others. Assessment of other cognitive functions such as language, spatial tasks, and executive functions is more difficult. It is often concluded that memory is a basic measure of a person's higher functions, when actually the situation is more complex. The term "cognition" comes from the Latin *cognitionem*, "a getting to know, acquaintance, knowledge," and can thus be used to refer to a complex assortment of mental functions. One difficulty in dealing with cognition is that it is so multifaceted: muscles contract and the heart pumps, but what, exactly, is cognition? It is involved in all of the higher functions of a person. In addition to the various forms of memory, the brain provides us with the joys and services of comprehension (understanding), language, calculation, orientation, perception, abstraction, route finding (finding our way around), judgment, spatial analysis, constructional abilities, anticipation, personality, behavior, social interactions, inhibition, and other abilities. (This is not to mention also the role of the brain in movement, blood pressure, heart rate, body temperature regulation, and countless other automatic activities.)

Comprehending cognition is challenging because the only thing we can use to understand our conscious mind is our conscious mind. You may know the joke about the fish being told about water and being unable to find it. Our eyes are made to look outward and not inward.

Intelligence or Intelligences?

The concept of intelligence is only a tool used in the shorthand of back-of-the-envelope understanding of the brain. There is clearly no single factor properly reflected in the term "intelligence," as demonstrated by the psychologist Martin Gardner in his book *Frames of Mind: The Theory of Multiple Intelligences*, first published in 1983. Memory is relatively easy to measure and is often thought to be the main sign of what is commonly called "intelligence." The ability to be creative and produce innovative ideas is more hidden. Emerson observed: "Indeed it is remarked that inventive men have bad memories. Sir Isaac Newton was embarrassed when the conversation turned on his discoveries and results; he could not recall them; but if he was asked why things were so or so he could find a reason on the spot."

Contrary to the belief of many, the various mental functions noted above do not work by themselves in isolation, and they are not the product of neurons working independently in different brain regions. The brain is magnificently interconnected – everything is connected to everything else. Some regions are connected more strongly and more quickly to certain other regions, but they are all connected. Studies of people whose corpus callosum, a large fiber tract connecting the right and left cerebral hemispheres, has been severed show that the right and left hemispheres have different skills: in most persons, the left having specialization for language and the right for social and visuo-spatial tasks. However, for those of us who have not had our corpus callosum sectioned, the two hemispheres are extensively connected to each other, so each has detailed information about what's happening on the other side. Similarly, although the temporal lobe near the middle of the brain (called the medial temporal lobe) is important for memory, the process of remembering is not located in that one area.

The cognitive aspects of daily life are accomplished through the complex interactions of the entire brain. All of our brain regions are dependent upon others, and none works alone. Our cognitive functions are the product of the whole brain and its ability to maintain a proper balance of interactions. These interfaces are both within the brain as well as between the brain and the rest of the body, the body's surroundings, and other persons. Sensory functions are particularly important. About 80 percent of the sensory input to the brain comes through the visual system, and audition is especially critical for communication. The senses of smell and taste have consistently declined in importance with evolution, although they are still relevant for many brain processes, not to mention the pleasure when walking into a bakery for the almond croissant you shouldn't be eating but you're going to eat anyway because it smells so enticing. Brain function can be altered when the sensory input the brain receives is disturbed. Many people with visual loss experience visual hallucinations of ghostly people and animals. Persons with severe hearing loss sometimes experience auditory hallucinations. A patient of mine with severe hearing loss, who did not have any cognitive deficits, frequently heard voices of friends and family members that weren't in the same room. This capacity of the sensory processing apparatus in the brain to provide a perception in the absence of input is not dependent upon any disturbance of consciousness or impairment of cognition. It is also well known that perfectly healthy people with good hearing and vision will develop hallucinations if exposed to severe sensory deprivation.

Changes in Memory and Cognition with Aging

Changes in cognitive function with age do not begin only in the later years of life. Researchers studying the performance of chess players found that performance improves rapidly until the age of 20 and peak performance is reached around the age of 35. Abilities deteriorate after 45 years of age.[46] Studies of healthy people have shown that memory function begins to decline from 30 years of age. Oxford University physician William Osler said that "the effective, moving, vitalizing work of the world is done between the ages of twenty-five and forty" and it was downhill from then on.[47] This view represents the long-standing and incorrect negative view of aging. Many declines are small, aren't noticeable, and don't happen to everyone. Numerous scientists, writers, and musicians produce insightful, creative work in later life. As you might imagine, changes are more marked in later life, especially after the age of 60. For most people these changes do not impact their quality of life or social or occupational functioning.

In aging there are commonly varying degrees of decline in cognitive function. These declines are not a disease in itself. I'm 72 years of age as I write this book. One day I was thinking about recommending *Moby-Dick; or, The Whale* to a friend and I couldn't recall the author's name. I tried as hard as I could to remember who wrote it, but had no idea. How could this be? I had known that *Moby-Dick* was written by Herman Melville since I was 14 years old and had known it since then. I had recently read about half of the book, found it ponderous, and gave up. The next day I tried again to remember Melville's name and failed. A week later, I tried again to remember the author of *Moby-Dick* and failed again. But somehow, I saw a picture of a friend in my mind while searching for the name. I wondered why I was seeing my friend Herman's image at a time like this. That image of my friend Herman helped me, of course, to realize that Herman Melville was the author I was looking for. I was concerned initially about this failure of memory but was reassured by the fact that I remembered what I had forgotten. My brain was working just fine. I'm just a little forgetful now and then, like most other people of a certain age. Had I been suffering from dementia, I would not have remembered what I had forgotten.

That said, it's unlikely that our memories will get better with age. Though wouldn't it be great if they did? There's this great line in Quentin Tarantino's film *Pulp Fiction* about memory. Two bandits are in a Los Angeles diner debating which crime they'll commit next. One is tired of robbing liquor stores, saying he'll never do it again. His girlfriend and partner-in-crime claims he says this every time, then asserts he'll forget about how much he hates robbing liquor stores in a day or two. He leans in, taps his finger on the table, and says, "The days of me forgetting are over. The days of me remembering have just begun."

In aging there are varying degrees of decline in cognitive function, which are quite common. These declines are not a disease in itself.

In aging there are varying degrees of decline in cognitive function, which are quite common. These declines are not a disease in itself. Aging is also associated with a profound increase in the risk of several neurodegenerative diseases such as Alzheimer's disease and Parkinson's disease. The effects of aging on performance in healthy people are dependent upon the functional capacity of the brain – they are not caused solely by brain changes with aging or solely by the development of brain disease. Performance is related to both pathology and functional capacity before the onset of disease. The same amount of age or disease-related brain changes may affect two people differently, based on their capacities beforehand. This is what is referred to as the cognitive reserve factor, also known as cognitive resilience (Chapter 2). It is a central focus of this book that we can enhance our reserve factors through our lifestyle choices.

The influences of aging and age-related disease (such as Alzheimer's disease) on brain function are determined

not only by the processes of aging and disease – the effect
of these processes on our performance ability depends
upon our cognitive, physical, psychological, and social
reserve factors. We all need to enhance these factors to
decrease the influence of aging processes on our function. Of course, we also wish to reduce the development
of age-related changes and reduce the risk of age-related
brain disease. We will be reviewing these opportunities in
Chapters 12–25.

Memory Has Many Forms

There are many forms of memory. This is important to
understand because many middle-age and older people
worry about memory loss. *Recent memory* involves episodes
occurring a short time ago, while *remote memory* is focused
on events that took place a longer time ago.

A fascinating aspect of *remote memory* is that it is difficult to evaluate. For example, the president of the United
States during most of World War II was Franklin Delano
Roosevelt. However, this is not necessarily a remote memory for many of us, since his name is still frequently mentioned in conversation and writing. (The East Side Highway
in New York City was named after Roosevelt.) Many of the
events in our early life which we recall are remembered
in part because we have been telling stories about them
for decades. Try remembering an event from a long time
ago you haven't told another person before. It is extremely
difficult! When the psychologist Jean Piaget was a child,
his nanny reportedly fought off a kidnapper. In return for
her bravery, his parents gave her a gold watch. Piaget often
recalled his memory of the dramatic event. Shortly before
her death, the nanny confessed that there had been no kidnapping attempt; she had manufactured the incident in
order to obtain a reward. Piaget's memory of the supposed
kidnapping, as convincing as it seemed, was false. He was

simply remembering the vividness of the non-event based on other people's stories. Many of our memories are not memories of events, but memories of memories. "It sometimes occurs that memory has a personality of its own, and volunteers or refuses its information at its will, not at mine," Emerson wrote in *Natural History of the Intellect*. "One sometimes asks himself, is it possible that it is only a visitor, not a resident?"

It is important to recognize that forgetting is a vital function of the brain and does not universally indicate the presence of disease.

When memory is a "visitor" and not a "resident," there may be several possible explanations. It is important to recognize that forgetting is a vital function of the brain and does not universally indicate the presence of disease. Life isn't like *Jeopardy!* It's not vital to intelligence to have automatic recall of random facts like the contestants on the popular television game show. It's more important to possess other, more complex forms of memory.

Let's discuss memory loss in people suffering from Alzheimer's disease. Persons with this disease often have a problem with memory that is limited to recent events, not events that happened years earlier. The reason for this is that a person with Alzheimer's disease has an impaired ability to make a memory of an event that happened three hours ago, not three years ago. This is called encoding, which is when the brain creates a memory trace. After the memory is encoded, it must be stored, and then recalled (retrieved). In Alzheimer's disease, there are impairments in all of the three processes of memory: encoding, storage, and retrieval. To remember something that happened a long time ago may depend primarily on retrieval and not upon encoding or storage, which may have taken place years ago before the onset of the disease.

Also, if I try to remember what I had for breakfast yesterday I'll probably fail to recall it, in large part because I
have never before tried to remember it, and I have never
spoken about it. However, if I try to recall something from
my earlier life, it may be that my memory of the event has
been well practiced over many years. Practice is incredibly
powerful for enhancing the power of memories. The last
thing that will be forgotten by a person with a progressive
memory deficit will likely be their first name, as it is the
most highly practiced word they have ever heard or spoken.

Episodic memory, or memory for events, and *procedural
memory*, memory of how to do something, are handled
by different systems in the brain. Alzheimer's disease
impairs episodic memory severely, but procedural memory is much less affected. Episodic memory relies upon
connections in the limbic system, which involves the hippocampus, and related structures in the temporal lobes.
Procedural memory involves the basal ganglia and cerebellum. There have been people with structural damage
to both right and left medial temporal lobes who have
severe deficits in episodic memory and cannot remember events from one moment to another. (This is pretty
much the plot of *Momento*, a Christopher Nolan movie
from 2000, about a man who relies on Polaroid photos
with handwritten notes on them to recall events in his
life.) However, people with poor memory for events (episodic memory) may have preserved memory for actions
(procedural memory) and be able to learn a new skill,
even though they are not able to remember that they
have been practicing the skill. It is shocking to see that a
person with advanced dementia may not recall that they
can play the piano, but still can sit at the keyboard and
play. An uncle of mine at 90 years of age had severe dementia from strokes and could not speak. When his wife

sang him a song from the 1940s he was able to hum along properly, to our great surprise.

In order for a memory to be retained it must be properly encoded. If this does not take place, memories may not be recalled and amnesia (*short-term memory loss*) may result. An amnestic person, who had no memory for recent events, can repeat a phone number to himself over and over and keep the number in his mind for a limited time, but once his rehearsal is interrupted, the memory is lost.

Consider how memory is tested; it is not enough to ask a person to remember something, then tell them what you would like them to remember, and then ask for their recall. It is necessary to be sure the person had an opportunity to encode the memory. If I ask a person to remember three objects and find that, five minutes later, they cannot recall the three objects, that may be a problem with memory – or it may be that they were not paying attention, didn't understand the task, or have a hearing problem.

Also, there needs to be an interval of distraction to prevent rehearsals, because *working memory* provides us with immediate recall, which allows very recent events to be briefly retained. (This is not actually a form of memory.) Working memory has been called the brain's sticky note, a tool for short-term storage (such as phone numbers, zip codes, or directions).

It is important to remember the importance of the role of attention in memory functioning (pun intended). A man accused of having a poor memory by his partner because he can't remember dinner plans for the weekend might not actually have a poor memory. He might suffer from memory impairment. But it may also be that he has a hearing problem or is not attentive. It may also be a result of a strategy in which the man has decided that what his partner is saying is not important. The Harvard psychologist

William James said, "The art of being wise is the art of knowing what to overlook." (Of course, the man's partner may beg to differ.)

"The art of being wise is the art of knowing what to overlook."

Knowing what to ignore reduces the demand on cognitive function. It is not uncommon for a person to become upset because a partner or spouse did not remember something. It may be that the person who appeared to be forgetful decided the item under discussion was not worth remembering. This can be a common event in which an apparent memory deficit is actually caused by an attentional decision (knowing what to overlook). Significant memory problems can also be caused by depression. If a person's mind is occupied by sad thoughts, it may be difficult to pay attention to life events.

The powerful influence of depression on memory is illustrated by this scenario. Imagine an 80-year-old woman who is grieving the death of her husband, six months earlier. She is asked to remember three things: "shoes, newspaper, and bus." She repeats the three items to the examiner, so it is clear that she heard them. She is then engaged in conversation briefly before being asked to recall the three objects. She says "shoes" but cannot recall the other two objects. This could be because of a brain disease such as Alzheimer's. It could also be because the word "shoes" reminds her that she had not yet decided what to do with her husband's shoes that are still tucked inside his closet. Her recall of her husband's shoes interfered with her memory of the other two objects. In this way her depression created memory impairment (see also Case Study 3).

Case Study 3

An 84-year-old former schoolteacher had slowly progressive memory loss for five years, with disorientation and severe impairment of recent memory. She had suffered from abdominal pains for over three decades, which could never be explained, even after many medical procedures. She reported that her abdominal pain was usually relieved at night when her husband massaged her feet. Shortly after she was diagnosed with Alzheimer's disease, she reported that her stomach pains indicated she was pregnant with twins. She had never previously had children. When I told her that her pregnancy was concerning because of her advanced age, she said, "That's right, doctor, I was worried about that myself. I am rather old to have a baby." The situation was quite stressful to her. Around the same time, she developed another delusion, reporting that she had two husbands, an older one who was with her constantly, and a younger one whom she hasn't seen in a while. Her husband reported that, in a restaurant, she asked him to take off their wedding ring because she was waiting for her other husband, a younger man, and he was going to be upset when he saw this older man wearing his wedding ring. I asked her which of her two husbands was the father of her babies.

"I don't know which one it was," she replied, "but I do remember that it was a good time."

This case illustrates the universal need for people to find an explanation for what happens to them. For over 30 years, her abdominal pain helped get the attention of her inattentive husband. When she became cognitively impaired, she developed a delusional pregnancy as her way of understanding her abdominal pain. Her failure of recent memory caused her to not recognize her aged husband, as she forgot that he had aged. At the same time, her memory of her husband as a younger man was relatively preserved, because it was an older memory from a time in which she was not impaired. It would have been better, of course, if the psychological issues associated with her long-standing abdominal pain had been dealt with before the onset of Alzheimer's disease.

In Order to Remember We Must Forget

I learned something critical about memory while talking to my daughter's third-grade class about the brain. We began by discussing all the things the brain does. The children raised their hands and offered the various functions of the brain very ably. One girl raised her hand and I asked her to answer the question, "What does the brain do?" She hesitated, apologized and said, "Oh, I forgot," indicating that she didn't remember what she wanted to say. I told her that she was right, and that she had a very valuable answer: that is, forgetting is a natural process and it is a function of the brain![48] If we try to remember everything – the name of every book we've read, every person in our neighborhood, every meal we've eaten, every pair of socks we have worn, every concert we've seen – our brains will become overburdened.

Our daily lives are much too complicated to remember everything that happens.

Our daily lives are much too complicated to remember everything that happens. The capacity of the brain is not infinite. A healthy mental life requires evaluation of life events and the selective retention in memory of things that need to be retained. Attention to these natural processes can help us understand changes in memory with aging. When I drive my car to the hospital every working day, I park in a multi-level-car-park concrete ramp, on the third, fourth, or fifth floors. There are times when I leave work at the end of the day and can't find my car. The reason may not be that I don't remember where I parked on that day. Rather, it may be that I hadn't forgotten where I parked the previous day. Some errors in memory such as this one are not errors in remembering, but errors in forgetting. The world is filled with irrelevant details, which do not demand our attention and which we should not be recalling. Imagine the demands on our memory capacities if we remembered everything that happened one morning: which socks we are wearing, which sock did we put on first, did we have fig jam or peanut butter on our toast, how much coffee did we drink, how much traffic was there on the drive to work, how many red or green lights did we encounter, who was with us in the elevator? The vast majority of events that happen to us are of no meaning and shouldn't be recalled.

Forgetting also enhances mental flexibility by removing information which is not of value. Imagine an airplane pilot making an approach to a runway, to land at night in a storm – hopefully the co-pilot is *not* saying, "Don't forget, captain, we have 156 passengers, 72 women and 64 men and 20 children, and 14,976 pounds of baggage." Forgetting can assist in the analysis of current situations by not burdening consciousness with past experiences which are not relevant to the matter at hand. The pilot landing at night in the storm will hopefully not be remembering the scene from the comedy movie *Airplane* in which a storm is mimicked.

Forgetting is an active process because it is necessary for learning. In forgetting, weaker connections of neurons and their synapses are removed. This strengthens the networks of neurons which we need for recall. Immune molecules and immune cells called microglia in the brain participate in this removal of weaker synapses that allows for remembering to take place. Exciting new research has shown that these molecules and cells in the brain that are critical for learning are influenced by the microbiota.[13] Thus, attention to the diet and lifestyle factors that influence the microbiota can enhance brain function.

The Importance of Attention, Perception, and Repetition

A key aspect of memory is attention, which is critically associated with perception. It will obviously be hard to remember something that we have not perceived. The world is made of countless stimuli, which one could try to pay attention to and recall. But this isn't possible; it exceeds the brain's processing capacity to pay attention to everything in the world. Because of this, we have evolved the capacity to make estimates and operate on these predictions, which are based on countless assumptions. So, if I hear the words "Joanna went to the library and came home with a most wonderful book," my brain will have predicted, unconsciously, that the word "book" was coming before the sentence was half over. This anticipatory process correctly predicted that Joanna did not pick up a lizard in the library, for example. This capacity for making assumptions is responsible for our ability to read, as well as our ability to process speech. Similarly, since I live in North America, if I see a small, furry animal in the trees near my house, I will assume it is a squirrel or chipmunk. I don't entertain the possibility of it being a baby monkey or a sloth. This assumption about what the animal in the tree is does not require my attention. If I see the animal in my peripheral vision, my brain will make the assumption unconsciously. When I am driving in the city, I pay attention to the car's position in the lane, its speed, the traffic signals and signs, and the pedestrians. But I cannot possibly pay attention to everything else, such as the signs of the stores, how many people are entering the stores, what pedestrians are wearing, whether the pedestrians are tall or short, whether the pedestrians are walking dogs, and, if so, what kind of dogs. All of these factors do not require my attention and must not occupy my attention if I am to be driving safely.

We all know that practice enhances memory.

What if I repeat that sentence?

We all know that practice enhances memory.

The unusual exact repetition of these seven words will enhance your memory of the sentence and the fact it represents. And if you go back and count to see if there really are seven words in each of the sentences and check that the sentences are perfectly identical, your memory of the sentence will be even greater. We learn through the enhancement of neuronal connections and the more we practice, the more the neural connections are enhanced, thereby improving memory.

Conclusion

In healthy people, their memory capacity and speed of learning declines with age, while their knowledge of events and words can increase. Older people have greater crystallized intelligence (knowledge, facts, and skills) than younger persons, and they may have more understanding of the environment. The result of long experience in aged people can produce wisdom, a factor balancing the losses of function.

Fortunately, there are things that we can do to enhance memory function with aging. These measures involve behavioral strategies, diet, exercise, mental activities, attention to medications, and consideration of the four multiple reserves.

5 THE NEURODEGENERATIVE DISEASES OF AGING

Considering everything, it seems we are dealing here with a special illness. An increasing number of similar cases have been observed during the last years.

This fact should persuade us not to be satisfied with classifying clinically undetermined cases by forcing them into the categories of recognized illnesses. There are certainly more psychiatric illnesses than are listed in our textbooks.

Translated from German from Alois
Alzheimer's original paper (1907)

Dementia and Alzheimer's Disease

What are the brain diseases most associated with aging? Alzheimer's disease is a good place to start. It is classified as a neurodegenerative disorder, which means that it is characterized by the progressive worsening and loss of structure and function in the nervous system. Only about 1 percent of Alzheimer's cases are caused by a defective gene. The most important risk factor for neurodegenerative disorders like Alzheimer's disease is age.

There is considerable misunderstanding about Alzheimer's disease and dementia. They are not the same thing. Let's begin with dementia. Dementia refers to a clinical syndrome (a group of symptoms which consistently occur together), with a loss of mental abilities, usually involving memory, visual–spatial functioning, language, perception, mood, behavior, and executive functions. Dementia almost always has a component of memory loss, especially memory for recent events. The word "dementia" is similar to the word "headache," in that the term "headache" does not indicate its cause. There are many causes of headache, and similarly there are many causes of dementia. Alzheimer's disease is the most common cause of the dementia syndrome.

It is important to recognize that the term "dementia" does not specify a diagnosis. The word "senile" only means "aged" and thus has no informative value whatsoever. A person having the onset of dementia before the age of 65 years may be referred to by some doctors as having "presenile dementia," but again, the term does not indicate the cause. It is also ageist and lacks meaning. The terms "senile," "senility," or "senile dementia" are obsolete and should not be used.

Every person with cognitive impairment needs a comprehensive evaluation to determine its cause. Since the terms "dementia," "presenile dementia," "senility," or "senile dementia" are not proper diagnoses, it is a sign of ignorance and negligence if a physician uses these words as a final diagnosis. These designations are descriptions of the symptoms and signs of an illness, and do not indicate the cause.

Alzheimer's Disease Statistics

The number of cases of Alzheimer's disease in the world is expected to double every 20 years because people are living longer (people over 85 years old are the fastest growing population in many middle-to-high-income countries). The prevalence and incidence of Alzheimer's disease doubles every five years after the age of 65. Because of this:

the average dementia-free 70-year-old man has about a 27 per cent probability of developing dementia during his life; and the average dementia-free 70-year-old woman has an estimated probability of 35 per cent of developing dementia.[49]

About 30–40 percent of people have Alzheimer's-related dementia at 90 years of age. Women have a higher risk of Alzheimer's disease, for reasons that are unclear.[50]

Alzheimer's disease is responsible for 60–80 percent of dementias. Other causes are Lewy body dementia, fronto-temporal lobar degeneration, Parkinson's dementia, and vascular cognitive impairment. It's common for many people with Alzheimer's disease also to have vascular changes in the brain, which include small and large strokes and bleeds and tissue damage associated with brain vessel disease. In the United States, studies have shown that the risk of Alzheimer's disease is perhaps twice as high in African Americans and 1.5 times higher in Hispanics, compared to white people.[51,52] This might be due to a higher prevalence of vascular disease, high blood pressure, obesity, and diabetes in these groups. In other parts of the world, Alzheimer's risk is lower in Africans and persons from India than in North America and Europe, perhaps because of high levels of physical exercise and low-fat, high-fiber diets in Africa and India.

The influence of social and economic factors is clear. Years of education are protective against the development of Alzheimer's disease, as was discussed previously in Chapter 2. The number of years of education, as well as the quality of education, is highly linked to economic factors worldwide. Education together with mental activities at home and at work form a crucial part of cognitive reserve.

What Are the Signs of Alzheimer's Disease?

Persons with Alzheimer's disease often have difficulties in several areas of cognitive function, including impairments in the following areas:

- recent memory, with relatively intact remote memory (recall of things that happened long ago)
- visual–spatial functions, which involve the analysis of what we see to understand relationships in space
- route-finding ability
- planning and anticipation
- abstraction, reasoning, decision making
- self-regulation
- attention
- control of behavior
- judgment
- emotional regulation
- word fluency

Many of the items on this list are referred to as executive functioning, higher-level skills we use for management of cognitive tasks and behaviors, and deficits are caused by difficulties in the frontal lobes (on top of your eyes) as well as the basal ganglia, thalamus, and temporal and parietal lobes. People with disturbed executive functioning will have trouble organizing activities, multitasking, word finding, and planning. They may be depressed, behave in a socially inappropriate way, or have a loss of interest in activities, poor recent memory, and poor understanding. People with executive-function changes often have poor insight into the nature of their deficits.

People with Alzheimer's disease may present in many different ways, but most commonly a loss of recent memory function is noted. The onset is usually gradual, and the disorder is consistently progressive. Changes with time are usually slow and the period from the onset of symptoms to death is about 10 years, but it is common for the duration to be either shorter or longer. The disease appears to be more aggressive in younger persons. The reason why the disease affects people in such different ways is largely unknown.

Mild cognitive impairment (MCI) describes a condition in which there is impaired cognition but no interference with social or occupational functioning. Persons with MCI are fully independent and have about a 50 percent chance of progressing to Alzheimer's disease in three years, and they may advance to have other conditions, including vascular cognitive impairment, Lewy body disease, and frontotemporal lobar degeneration. There are also persons with MCI who improve and do not progress to dementia. Mild cognitive impairment describes a level of impairment which is intermediate between normal function and dementia. People with MCI have memory impairment which can be documented, a complaint by the individual or family member, normal activities of daily living, no decline in social or occupational functioning, and generally normal cognitive functions otherwise, without dementia. There also are also forms of MCI which do not primarily involve memory loss.

It is often believed that persons with Alzheimer's disease are not aware of their illness. This is not correct. People will often have the concern that they have it – and they may be correct. There are also many people who believe they have it who do not have Alzheimer's disease or any other serious problem. Although many people with this disease may be aware of their deficits, many others are unaware of the nature and extent of their disability. This denial may unfortunately limit their access to proper evaluation and treatment. It is best to do whatever is necessary to have them come in to have a workup – it may be a matter of life and death.

Persons with Alzheimer's disease are at an increased risk of delirium, which causes significant cognitive impairment, along with a fluctuating level of consciousness, often with hallucinations (perceptions of an unreal nature) and delusions (false beliefs). Delirium is often associated with systemic illness, as well as the effects of drugs. Delirium provides a good example of the importance of maintaining a proper balance of the four reserve factors. For example, an 80-year-old person with the early stages of Alzheimer's disease may be doing very well at home but, if the person experiences major life changes (death of a spouse or change in medications), delirium may result. Possible physical reserve factors that may interact with Alzheimer's disease to cause delirium include kidney impairment, urinary tract infection, respiratory difficulty, pneumonia, anemia, pain, constipation, and other factors, as well as medications. The development of delirium is an important indication that there is some critical physical problem going on, which must be remedied quickly. Psychological and social reserve factors can also be involved in triggering delirium, such as grief, depression, loss of friends, loss of mobility, isolation, and financial stress.

Alzheimer's First Case

In order to understand what happens in the brain in Alzheimer's disease it helps to learn about the first case. The disease was first reported in 1907 by Alois Alzheimer, a Bavarian neuropsychiatrist. Alzheimer was devoted to the study of the cerebral origins of behavioral diseases. The commonest of these conditions at that time was neurosyphilis. Alzheimer studied pathology with Karl Weigert, developer of early staining techniques for bacteria and the brain. As a young clinician, Alzheimer was asked to accompany a wealthy syphilitic patient and his wife on a tour of Egypt. Following their arrival, the patient died, and Alzheimer accompanied the widow, Nathalie Geisenheimer, home. He later married her; she supported his research career with her own resources. Alzheimer was an excellent teacher in small groups, but a poor lecturer. His students loved him because of the personal attention he gave them and his excellent sense of humor. At the end of every day there would be a cigar butt of Alzheimer's next to every microscope in the lab.

Alzheimer had a female patient named Auguste Deter who presented with severe memory loss and word-finding problems at the age of 51. She also had delusions (false beliefs) and accused her husband of having an affair. After she died, aged 55, Alzheimer studied her brain. It showed that she didn't suffer from neurosyphilis (a common cause of behavioral problems at the time). Her brain showed the accumulation of fibrillar (like a fiber) material inside neurons, later called neurofibrillary tangles. Alzheimer presented his findings about Deter's brain at a meeting of the Southwest German Alienists Association in 1906 (alienist is a nineteenth-century word for psychiatrist). Alzheimer's talk at the meeting was the only one that did not elicit any discussion (the Swiss psychiatrist Carl Jung also spoke that day). It is likely that the audience didn't know what to say about Alzheimer's report.

Alzheimer did not consider Auguste Deter's problem to be distinct from the more common occurrence of dementia in older persons, which at the time was referred to as senile dementia or senile psychosis. However, because of academic rivalry, Alzheimer's chief, Emil Kraepelin (1856–1926, Director of the Royal Psychiatric Clinic in Munich where Alzheimer worked) named the disease after Alzheimer in 1910, in his textbook of psychiatry, and specified it as occurring in younger people, to distinguish it from the more common disorder of the aged. Kraepelin was the leading psychiatrist in the world at that time and his textbook was the foremost work in the field for several decades. Kraepelin wished to have the honor given to the German member of his group in Munich, and not to the Czech's Arnold Pick or Oskar Fischer, who were doing similar work in the field. Weigert, Fischer, Pick, and Alzheimer's wife were all Jewish. Kraepelin's antisemitism may have also played a role in his choice of Alzheimer for the eponym.[53]

Alzheimer's Disease Misperceptions

After Alzheimer's 1907 report, the subject of dementia received little attention. This is because of the false belief that dementia was commonly caused in older persons by "hardening of arteries in the neck," also referred to as atherosclerosis of the carotid arteries. For most of the twentieth century, the terms for what we now call Alzheimer's disease were organic brain syndrome, senile psychoses, senile dementia, senility, and arteriosclerotic brain disease. It is true that dementia can be caused by cerebrovascular disease, but Alzheimer's disease is a much more common cause. This error was compounded by the finding, in 1951, of Seymour Kety and colleagues at the National Institutes of Health in Bethesda, Maryland, that people with what was then called the "psychoses of senility" had reduced blood flow to the brain.[54] These errors contributed to a relative lack of interest in Alzheimer's. Later, Kety's group showed that the reduced blood flow was a result – not the cause – of the diminished use of oxygen and glucose.

Until the 1970s, Alzheimer's disease was thought to be rare and caused by a problem with blood vessels in the brain. And since there were no good treatments for vessel diseases, researchers and doctors didn't worry about it too much. Widespread sexism may have also played a role in this bias, as there are many more older women than older men. In the United States, at 85 years of age and older, there are 187 women for every 100 men (2017). Dr. Alyson McGregor's 2020 book, *Sex Matters: How Male-Centric Medicine Endangers Women's Health – and What We Can Do About It*, reviews how the lack of medical research on women has influenced their healthcare. Today we know that Alzheimer's disease isn't rare. It is quite common. We also know that Alzheimer's is a disease of neurons, not of blood vessels.

Alzheimer's first case died at the age of 55, but the more common occurrence of dementia in people over the age of 65 was largely ignored for the 70 years after Alzheimer's original report. Neurologist Robert Katzman at the Albert Einstein College of Medicine in New York noted in 1976 that early-onset (occurring before the age of 65 years) and late-onset dementias with neurofibrillary tangles and senile plaques were similar and were probably the same disease. In his paper, "The prevalence and malignancy of Alzheimer disease: a major killer," Katzman pointed out that the main risk factor for the disease was aging, and that global populations were getting older at a rapid rate, indicating correctly that the disease was to become a major, worldwide problem.[55]

It is never normal for an aged person to have a failure of memory that significantly interferes with everyday life.

Is it normal for older people to have significant memory disabilities? No. It is never normal for an aged person to have a failure of memory that significantly interferes with everyday life. As we have discussed earlier, memory function declines with aging but age-related forgetfulness does not influence completion of the tasks of daily life, as discussed in Chapter 4.

What Goes Wrong in the Brain in Alzheimer's Disease?

In order to understand what can be done to delay or prevent the development of Alzheimer's disease, it helps to know about the nature of the brain changes that occur. A brain affected by Alzheimer's disease has several abnormalities. There is a loss of brain substance in the cortex where the neurons reside, referred to as atrophy. There are also neurofibrillary tangles, deposits in cells of an aggregated (clumped) protein called tau. The tangles are accompanied by larger deposits, called plaques, between cells of the amyloid-beta protein, which is also aggregated. Scientists believe these two fibrillar proteins damage neurons and cause inflammation and the death of neurons. It has also been found in Alzheimer's disease that the supporting cells of the brain, called glia, become hyperactive. It is not known if this inflammatory reaction is in response to these deposits, or if it is contributing to their development (or perhaps both, at different times in the development of the disease). There are also deposits of the amyloid-beta protein in blood vessels, causing damage to the circulation, resulting in diminished blood flow and, at times, small and large brain hemorrhages. The disease is accompanied by excessive amounts of free radicals – products of the metabolism of oxygen and glucose, which impair proteins, lipids, carbohydrates, and DNA and are central to the disease process. This process is called oxidative toxicity.

In 1985, George Glenner and his colleagues at the National Institutes of Health made a major breakthrough when they discovered the amino acid sequence of the protein at the core of the plaques. Using this information, researchers learned that the protein, now called amyloid beta, was made by a gene on chromosome 21, called the amyloid precursor protein (APP). This explains why people with Down syndrome nearly always develop the behavioral and structural abnormalities of Alzheimer's disease after the ages of 30–40; they have three copies of the APP gene and, as a result, they make 50 percent more of the protein than people without Down syndrome. This information about the structure of the amyloid-beta protein and its parent protein, APP, helped geneticists in London and elsewhere to identify mutations responsible for the development of early-onset Alzheimer's disease (see Chapter 11).

Protein Deposits and Protein Folding

Research over the past two decades using molecular biology and brain imaging with positron emission tomography has shown that the earliest change in the brain in Alzheimer's is the deposition of amyloid beta in the cortex. This is followed later by the tau deposits, and then by cortical atrophy (loss of substance of the cortex). It is only after this process has been active in the brain for 10–20 years does notable cognitive impairment develop. It is now clear that the development of Alzheimer's disease is a very chronic process, which begins many years before the first symptoms or signs. The good news is that because the progress of the brain changes are so slow we have an opportunity to delay their progress through attention to our four reserve factors, particularly our activities and diet.

The good news is that because the progress of the brain changes are so slow we have an opportunity to delay their progress through attention to our four reserve factors, particularly our activities and diet.

Alzheimer's is a disease of proteins. Proteins are made in the cytoplasm of cells out of a sequence of building blocks, called amino acids, which are determined by the cell's DNA. When proteins are made, they do not have a three-dimensional structure. In order for the protein to work it must adopt a correct structure. This can be a helix, similar to one of the two strands of the structure of DNA, or other coiled forms. Parts of the molecule fold onto other parts of the protein, giving it a precise three-dimensional configuration. The acquisition of this correct structure is referred to as protein folding. It is critical that proteins adopt the correct structure; if the proper structure is not generated, the protein may be non-functional and may also be toxic. Errors in the structure of proteins are called misfolding and are key to understanding Alzheimer's disease.

Every cell has a protein-folding quality-control mechanism, which evaluates the process and recycles the amino acids of proteins which are not properly folded. Proteins can be folded into a cross-beta-pleated sheet, in which regions of the molecule are folded tightly upon each other in a very highly stable assembly that is resistant to destruction. Proteins that fold with a large amount of beta-pleated sheet are referred to as amyloid proteins. The silk of a spider's web is one example of an amyloid protein. Because of the tight bonding of segments of the silk protein to itself the silk of a spider's web is perhaps the strongest substance in the world, in consideration of its very low mass. The word amyloid does not refer to a specific protein, but to its unique three-dimensional structure.

Amyloid structures have the important characteristic of having a potentially "transmissible" nature. One amyloid protein can cause an identical or similar protein to adopt an amyloid configuration. Proteins that have the ability to cause transformation of other proteins to a similar structure are referred to as prions (proteinaceous infectious agents), a term coined by the Nobel Prize-winning neurologist Stanley Prusiner. The infectivity of these agents means that the abnormal protein configuration can be transmitted internally – from one region of the body to another, and from one part of the brain to another. However, someone with Alzheimer's disease, Parkinson's disease, or amyotrophic lateral sclerosis (ALS) cannot transmit the disease to another person.

Protein-folding quality control is especially critical for the brain because neurons are among the most long-lived cells in the body. Liver cells are replaced throughout life, but neurons are mostly non-dividing and are present from birth. Because of this, neurons have greater vulnerability to the accumulation of damage associated with misfolded proteins. It has become apparent in the last 10 years that the proteins deposited in the brain in Alzheimer's disease, Parkinson's disease, and ALS have amyloid characteristics which are transmissible from one body part to another, and in some occasions from one animal to another. This process is believed to be responsible for the transmission of abnormally folded proteins from the gut to the brain and from the nose to the brain. It has been proposed that this is how the disease process in neurodegeneration is initiated[56,57] (see Figure 5). Knowing about these disease mechanisms helps us to understand the measures we can take to both lower our risk of these diseases and enhance our resistance to their brain changes. The dietary measures reviewed in Chapter 20 may help lower the rate of protein misfolding in the brain, through the actions of the gut bacteria.

Inflammation in Alzheimer's Disease

It is important to appreciate the role of inflammation in Alzheimer's disease because of the ways we can influence its activities, through our attention to the multiple reserves. Inflammation involves both innate immunity (a rapid first response from circulating and brain immune cells) and adaptive immune systems (slower long-term memory responses that may be lifelong). Brain cells called microglia enforce immune surveillance, monitoring the environment for disease-causing factors such as viruses or toxins. The microglia also assist in establishing connections between neurons (synapse formation), provide growth factors, and

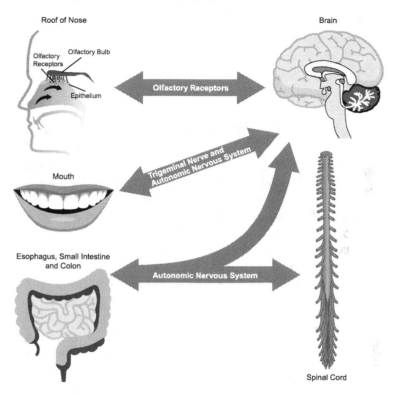

Figure 5 Pathways from gut to brain and brain to gut
Gut microbial factors in the intestines, mouth, throat, and nose can influence the brain and spinal cord though the autonomic nervous system and the cranial nerves. The autonomic nervous system is an important part of our control systems, which acts mostly without consciousness, and manages body functions, such as heart rate, digestion, intestinal movement, breathing, urination, and sexual function. These pathways can work in both directions. Agents transferred through these routes can include microbes, proteins, and other molecules. The circulation may also be a route of transfer. (Reproduced from reference 56.)

destroy unneeded cells and synapses. They also monitor the production and clearance of brain proteins.

The activities of the immune system can also be divided into resistance and tolerance functions. (Both of these aspects of the immune system involve innate and adaptive features.) Resistance protects us from disease by battling microbial growth and spread. Tolerance provides limits to disease without changing the growth of microbes.[58,59] We need the immune system to protect us from overgrowth of microbes; this is the resistance activity. At the same time, we need the immune system to tolerate microbes that are present on our surfaces and in our body cavities. As you will see in Chapter 8 on the microbiota, these organisms are necessary for life and they must be tolerated. The microbial contents inside us have evolved the capacity to enhance this tolerance. Thus, our immune processes are heavily influenced by microbial factors. These functions influence the nature of our reserve capacity because of their effects on the brain's response to age-related changes. An 80-year-old person who has been developing amyloid-beta plaques, as well as deposits of other aggregated proteins, in the brain for 15 years may be better off if the amyloid deposits are tolerated, as opposed to being aggressively targeted by the immune system. There is evidence to suggest that the immune response to age-related brain changes may be damaging. And our diet may influence the development of this tolerance.

Can We Influence the Development of the Alzheimer's Process in the Brain?

A critical element in this discussion is the fact that our lifestyle behaviors influence these processes, including protein misfolding, free radical production, and inflammation. The cellular protein-folding quality-control mechanism can be overwhelmed and become less effective if the body is stressed by free radicals or there is an excessive production of misfolded proteins. And the transmission and initiation of amyloid formation is related to diet. Free radicals in the brain are also affected by what we eat. Physical and mental exercise also has protective effects against the development of Alzheimer's disease. The many interactions of lifestyle behaviors and the processes in this disease are reviewed in Chapters 12–25. A key message is that (a) there are behaviors (things that we do) that influence the diseases themselves, and also (b) our behaviors influence how we're affected by disease if it does develop. Both pathways (a) and (b) are influenced by the multiple reserve factors.

A key message is that (a) there are behaviors (things that we do) that influence the diseases themselves, and also (b) our behaviors influence how we're affected by disease if it does develop. Both pathways (a) and (b) are influenced by the multiple reserve factors.

Physical and mental activities help produce growth factors in the brain that enhance cognitive reserve. This helps delay the progress of the Alzheimer's process in the brain and also enhances the brain's resistance to behavior changes caused by this process. Similar relations can be proposed for dietary measures as well, as discussed in Chapter 20.

Who Should Be Consulted for the Diagnosis and Care of Persons with Dementia?

Physicians and nurse practitioners in the domains of neurology, psychiatry, geriatrics, and family medicine can all provide this important evaluation. What is critical is that the provider has experience and interest in this area. Unfortunately, for financial reasons, widespread commitment on the part of universities, hospitals, and other institutions to provide this comprehensive evaluation and intervention is lacking in many locations. A thorough mental status examination involving standardized testing is advisable, occasionally including a battery of tests administered by a neuropsychologist. Symptoms similar to those in Alzheimer's disease can also be caused by anemia or leukemia, indicating the need for a complete blood count. Liver and kidney diseases may also cause brain dysfunction mimicking Alzheimer's disease, suggesting the need for a complete metabolic panel. Thyroid deficiency and excess can also cause marked memory problems and vitamin B12 deficiency is an important cause of treatable dementia. High total plasma homocysteine levels have been associated with an increased risk of Alzheimer's disease and stroke; such high levels are also associated with the deficiency of vitamins B12, B6, and folic acid, which can be corrected with supplementation. If there is rapid progression of onset before the age of 60 years, it may be necessary to test also for HIV and syphilis serology, and to carry out an electroencephalogram (EEG), lumbar puncture, and other measures. Neuroimaging of the brain with computed tomography or magnetic resonance imaging are needed in every case for comprehensive evaluation. Every person with impaired memory or a suspicion of Alzheimer's disease should be evaluated by a medical professional who is experienced and interested in this problem.

Every person with impaired memory or a suspicion of Alzheimer's disease should be evaluated by a medical professional who is experienced and interested in this problem.

The accuracy of the diagnosis of Alzheimer's disease can be verified in many cases through the tests and evaluations noted above, with a diagnostic certainty of 80–90 percent. This may be improved with the addition of amyloid scanning with positron emission tomography (PET), or from a spinal tap with analysis of cerebrospinal fluid levels of the Alzheimer-associated proteins. Recently, tests for Alzheimer-related molecules in the blood have been shown to be highly sensitive and specific for the disease. Tests may improve the diagnostic certainty to more than 95 percent in some cases. The indication for these tests is related to the person's age. In persons greater than 70 years of age, these tests are of lesser value, because findings suggestive of Alzheimer's disease may indicate that the person will develop the disease if they live to be 80 years or older, and not necessarily that the disease is the cause of their impairment at the time the test is completed. At the age of 85, there are three times as many people with signs of developing Alzheimer's disease in the brain without dementia than those who have the disease with dementia.[60]

Friends and family members of an older person with significant memory difficulties often assume the loved one must have Alzheimer's disease and that there is nothing to be done. This is a serious and dangerous error, as many older people with dementia have a treatable and reversible condition. It is common that older persons are taking the wrong drugs in the wrong combinations and develop memory problems which are completely reversible. Similarly, older people may have unrecognized depression and, with appropriate therapy or medication, their lives improve. Every person who is having significant memory problems, regardless of age, requires evaluation by an appropriately experienced healthcare worker.

Risk and Protective Factors for Alzheimer's Disease

Risk factors for Alzheimer's disease include age, female gender, head injury, high-fat diet, smoking, alcohol abuse, hypertension, depression, diabetes, lack of physical activity, lack of mental demands at work, lack of mental demands during recreational activities, low levels of education, and obesity. Many of these factors are modifiable and actions can diminish their influence. Vascular risk factors are particularly important; these include: hypertension, coronary artery disease, atrial fibrillation, sleep apnea, depression, congestive heart failure, hyperlipidemia, obesity, and diabetes mellitus. Hypertension in midlife is particularly linked to late development of Alzheimer's disease.[61] Improved blood pressure control has been recommended to decrease the occurrence of the disease. Because of the relatively late onset of most cases of Alzheimer's disease, delaying the onset to a later age may mean that many people do not live long enough to develop the disease. If the onset age was delayed by five years, the prevalence of the disease could be cut in half. It is estimated that as many as 33–50 percent of worldwide cases of Alzheimer's disease may be attributable to potentially modifiable risk factors.[62] Midlife cognitive activity is associated with a lower risk of Alzheimer's disease as well as slower cognitive decline.[16,17,63] Ways to diminish disease risk and decrease rate of progression are noted in Chapters 12–25.

Because of the relatively late onset of most cases of Alzheimer's disease, delaying the onset to a later age may mean that many people do not live long enough to develop the disease.

Treatments for Alzheimer's Disease

Genetic studies have uncovered several important metabolic pathways that are involved in Alzheimer's disease in its inherited forms. This work has led to the development of experimental therapies, which are currently under evaluation. Unfortunately, the last 20 years of clinical trials of these approaches have not been rewarding. A large problem in this area is that there are no animal models for non-genetic Alzheimer's disease, which is found in 99 percent of human cases. Because of this, most animal research has involved mice with genetic abnormalities that 99% of patients do not have. Persons with Alzheimer's disease may be treated with cholinesterase inhibitors and glutamate receptor blockers. These medications may improve memory and general behavior in some of them, but only to a small degree.[64] Side effects of these agents include a slowed heart rate, nausea, vomiting, and difficult sleep. Antidepressants may also help at times.[64] Genes and clinical trials are discussed in Chapters 11 and 23.

On June 7, 2021, the US Food and Drug Administration approved the monoclonal antibody aducanumab (Aduhelm) for the treatment of Alzheimer's disease. The agent was developed to bind to the amyloid-beta protein in the brain. PET scans demonstrated the effective removal of the deposits from the brain. However, the change in cognitive decline over time associated with the treatment was minor. Also, over 40% suffered potentially serious brain swelling following the infusion. Furthermore, in November 2020, prior to the ultimate FDA approval, an FDA scientific advisory panel recommended, with a vote of 10 to 0, that the agent should not be approved. The developer of the antibody, Biogen, announced an annual price of $28,000 for the agent. Consequently, several leading medical centers have announced that they will not be prescribing the agent because of the high cost, small amount of improvement in the subjects' functions, and the risk of side effects. I will also not be prescribing the drug for these reasons and will recommend that rather than taking an agent which is known not to be effective, and potentially risky, patients should participate in clinical trials of other therapies. Participation in a clinical trial could possibly allow a person to receive a truly effective agent.

Treatable and Potentially Reversible Dementia

It is not uncommon that persons suspected of having Alzheimer's disease have an illness which is potentially reversible (see Case Study 4). A comprehensive evaluation carried out by a physician interested in and experienced with the disease must be completed. The top three possibilities for reversible or treatable dementia are polypharmacy (drug effects), depression, and systemic toxic-metabolic conditions. Drugs can commonly cause cognitive impairment in older persons. This important topic is addressed in Chapter 23. Depression can also cause cognitive impairment, even in persons who are not aware that they are depressed. A wide range of systemic toxic-metabolic conditions can also cause cognitive loss. These conditions include disorders of every organ system of the body. A list of just a few of these conditions includes anemia, B12 deficiency, B1 deficiency, leukemia, kidney failure, malabsorption, congestive heart failure, urinary tract infection, hypothyroidism and other endocrine disorders, subdural hematoma (a form of brain bleeding), HIV/AIDS, and chronic obstructive pulmonary disease. Because these conditions can cause cognitive problems that mimic Alzheimer's disease, it is necessary to perform screening blood tests to document their absence. There is no age at which dementia is normal.

There is no age at which dementia is normal.

Frontotemporal Lobar Degeneration

Frontotemporal lobar degeneration (FTLD) (previously called Pick's disease) is a neurodegenerative disorder which mostly affects the frontal and temporal lobes of the brain. FTLD is frequently seen with onset before the age

Case Study 4

A 76-year-old man presented to my cognitive disorders clinic with a chief complaint of forgetfulness that was of gradual onset and slowly progressive. He had been forgetting days of the week and other recent events for the past two years. His forgetting did not interfere with his activities of daily living, however. Because of his forgetfulness he preferred to spend most of his days in bed. He had poor sleep and frequent awakenings, as well as depression following the death of his stepson in a car accident. There was no family history of neurological or psychiatric illnesses. On examination, he was disoriented about the date, could not recall any of five objects after two minutes, could not copy a cube, and incorrectly drew the hands on the clock.

It turned out that the man was prescribed two drugs that can depress the function of the central nervous system, diazepam and hyoscyamine. Diazepam is a sedative and is metabolized slowly, with a plasma half-life of over 30 hours. This means that it takes 30 hours after a dose of the medication for the plasma level to fall by half. Thus, a daily dose, taken every 24 hours, will result in too much of the drug in the bloodstream. The patient was advised to stop taking these two drugs. Hyoscyamine is a drug known to interfere with neurotransmission in the brain, especially in older persons. Gradual withdrawal of the two drugs over one month was recommended. My initial diagnosis was that his gradual decline in cognition was caused by diazepam and hyoscyamine toxicity.

When he returned to my office two months later, he was no longer taking either medication. As a result, he had recovered and performed normally on mental status tests. He was no longer spending the day in bed and was participating in his previous activities. This is a case of treatable, reversible dementia. Every patient deserves a comprehensive evaluation to see if a causative factor can be found that created a reversible condition. In 2020, colleagues and I described this case in the journal *Neurology*.[65]

In 1989, I published a similar case in the *Journal of the American Medical Association*.[66] A 74-year-old woman came to me with what also turned out to be a treatable dementia. I referred to the process of uncovering such cases as the "saga of the treatable dementias." To the Vikings of historic Norway, the word "saga" was a word meant to describe a "heroic narrative." I felt that this was a good way to indicate that the search for treatable dementias requires tenacity and ferocity.

of 65 and causes different behavioral abnormalities than Alzheimer's disease.

People with FTLD may develop one of three clinical pictures:

difficulty speaking, with trouble finding words, usually leading to stuttering speech, called primary progressive aphasia;

a pattern called "behavioral variant" in which there is a lack of inhibition (disinhibition), where persons say things that are hurtful and inappropriate, often accompanied by rude sexual behaviors, excessive and unreasonable spending, and unusual appetites (see Case Study 5); and

a form of cognitive loss called semantic dementia in which there is a progressive loss of knowledge and of the meaning of words.

The behavioral problems in FTLD usually are of slow onset, with a gradual progression, and often include delusions and hallucinations, sleeping disorders, and poor money management. FTLD can be frequently identified by the pattern of atrophy on scans of the brain. In Alzheimer's disease, atrophy is usually widespread, although it may be worse in the parietal lobes and hippocampus. In FTLD, the atrophy is most often enhanced in the frontal and temporal lobes. There are several genes that have been identified as causing FTLD. These genetic forms of FTLD are of early onset and autosomal dominant. Motor neuron disease, also called ALS, may occur together with FTLD, either early or late in the disease process.

Recently, it's been reported that more years of education is associated with slower loss of brain substance and cognitive impairment in persons with FTLD of genetic origin. This illustrates that even when there is a disease-causing gene, personal life choices can influence the expression of brain disease. Strategies for adjusting lifestyle behaviors are reviewed in the applications section of the book, Chapters 12–25.

Case Study 5

I had a patient who was a 72-year-old man. He went with his wife to pick up clothes at a dry cleaner. After paying, he asked the young woman working there if she would like to go out to have a cup of coffee with him after work. She said, "absolutely not." His wife asked him why he had approached this woman, considering the fact that they had been married for over 40 years.

"She's a hot chick," he said. "I'm a sexy old man. What's wrong with that?"

The man had also been involved in recent car accidents. He'd been driving erratically and at excessive speed with poor reasoning for the past several years. He was "ranting and raving" at times because he said his wife refused to share her innermost thoughts with him. He became suspicious of her and spent $600 on tickets for a rock concert. (An excessive amount based on past spending patterns.) He told a nurse in the clinic that he was a "horny old man." He called 911 to say that his wife was hitting him in the back with a baseball bat. (Not true.) He was also forgetful and accusatory toward his wife and didn't often bathe. On a trip to China, he refused to get into his group's car in the Hong Kong airport and took a separate taxi, because he was afraid that he would be kidnapped.

He did not have any family history of neurological or psychiatric conditions. When he was examined in clinic, he was shown a random photograph from a magazine advertisement of a young woman and asked to describe the picture. He proceeded to provide inappropriate details about her body. On exam he had trouble with idioms, yet his memory was relatively intact. Looking at a picture of a shirt, all he could see were the buttons. He called a pigeon a duck and could only name three words beginning with the letter F. A PET scan of glucose metabolism in the brain showed diminished glucose use in the right frontal and temporal lobes and magnetic resonance imaging showed loss of brain substance in the anterior temporal and frontal regions. His behavioral problems were difficult to manage, and despite trial of several medications, he needed to be admitted to a nursing home. This form of frontotemporal dementia, called behavioral variant, has no known cause in the cases that are not inherited. The treatment options for the behavioral abnormalities are poor. Luckily, this syndrome is relatively uncommon.

Parkinson's and Lewy Body Diseases

In 1817, British physician James Parkinson described a disorder of slow onset and gradual progression. Parkinson's disease is characterized by these signs:

- slow resting tremor;
- slowness of movement;
- rigidity (resistance to passive motion); and
- postural instability.

The disorder is associated with an abnormal accumulation in the brain of fibrillar deposits of the neuronal protein alpha-synuclein, called Lewy bodies. These deposits are thought to be the cause of damage to the motor system of the brain, particularly in a central region called the midbrain, which is critical for coordinating motor abilities. In many cases, these deposits can extend to other regions of the brain, aside from the midbrain, and cause dementia. In Parkinson's disease, there are deposits of alpha-synuclein, associated with elevated inflammatory molecules and oxidative stress in the plasma and cerebrospinal fluid. In some cases, dementia develops, followed by motor features, which is called Lewy body disease. The presence of the motor features of Parkinson's disease is often called "parkinsonism."

Autosomal-dominant genes can cause Parkinson's disease in about 10 percent of cases and several other genes may influence the risk without being clearly causative. The heritability of Parkinson's disease is estimated at about 27 percent.[67] Healthy aging is associated with some features of motor impairment, but not with the full spectrum of manifestations seen in Parkinson's disease. Healthy older persons may have a faster tremor that becomes more active with movement, called essential tremor, as opposed to the slower tremor seen in Parkinson's disease, which is usually more marked at rest. The risk of this disease is increased by repetitive head injury, and metal and pesticide exposure. Growing up on a farm is associated with a higher risk of development of Parkinson's disease. Cerebrovascular risk factors, such as stroke, hypertension, and heart disease are also associated with the disease, an effect similar to their association with Alzheimer's disease.[68] Low levels of physical activity and not smoking are also risk factors for the disease. Although it has been established that non-smokers have a higher risk of Parkinson's disease than smokers it is certainly advisable to not smoke. The risk of serious negative consequence of smoking (e.g., cancer, emphysema, stroke) are much more significant than the lower risk of the disease in smokers. Exercise has been noted to improve the movement disability as well as the rate of cognitive decline seen in persons with Parkinson's disease.

Genes that are linked to Parkinson's disease have recently been discovered, which are involved in immune function, suggesting a role of the immune system in the illness. The clumping of the alpha-synuclein molecule may begin in neurons in the gut, early in life. The pathological process may be transmitted from the gut to the brain by way of the gut–brain axis (see Figure 5). There is early onset of constipation and loss of the sense of smell in Parkinson's disease, sometimes beginning more than a decade before the onset of motor findings. It is believed that these changes are due to the damage to olfactory neurons in the nose, causing loss of the ability to smell, and impairment of neurons in the gut, causing constipation. People who have had the neuronal pathway from the gut to the brain (the vagus nerve) severed early in life have been found to have a lower risk of developing Parkinson's disease later, supporting the theory that the problem is beginning in the gut. Work done in our labs, as well as in the California Institute of Technology in Los Angeles, strongly suggest that the microbiota are involved in Parkinson's disease.[56,57]

The motor features of Parkinson's disease can be well controlled through medication for many years. However, after about 10 years, the impact of medications decline. For some patients, deep brain stimulation through implanted electrodes may be helpful. At present, the dementia that occurs in Parkinson's or Lewy body disease cannot be reversed by any disease-modifying medications. Some patients may gain improvement from acetylcholinesterase inhibitors.

The same four reserve factors that may help to alter the course of Alzheimer's disease are also relevant in Parkinson's disease. A physically active lifestyle with a diet that inhibits excess inflammation is desirable.

Amyotrophic Lateral Sclerosis (ALS)

A 56-year-old friend of mine, who was a bodybuilder, living in Japan, developed weakness in his hands, which was rapidly progressive over one year. Neurological examination showed weakness in both arms with twitching of muscle fibers under the skin, and a diagnosis of ALS was made. His weakness progressed until he could not use his arms in any way, although he could walk and speak. Difficulty swallowing developed, and he died of ALS when food became lodged in his throat after four years of illness. Another person with ALS is a 54-year-old pilot who had progressive weakness of swallowing and speaking caused by ALS until he was unable to eat or talk, although he could still swim and use a computer. He is fed through a feeding tube and is developing weakness in his limbs. In both cases, there was no family history of ALS and there is no very effective disease-modifying therapy. These cases demonstrate the profound cruelty of the disease.

ALS is another neurodegenerative disorder which is caused by autosomal-dominant genes in about 10 percent of cases. Risk factors for ALS include the following:[69]

- genes (it is estimated that about 60 percent of the risk of developing ALS is genetic);
- age;
- smoking;
- exposure to toxins (lead, manganese, or pesticides);
- head injury (football, soccer, exposure to explosions); and
- low intake of antioxidants and polyunsaturated fatty acids.

The disease causes progressive weakness and loss of muscle mass throughout the body, with death usually developing within three years from diagnosis. In ALS there is a shrinkage and loss of motor neurons in the brain and spinal cord and deposition of abnormally folded neuronal proteins as well as inflammation. Also found in ALS is the presence of peripheral immune cells in the brain with activated inflammatory molecules. Persons with ALS may develop dementia after the initial onset of motor difficulties. Sadly, persons with FTLD may later develop signs of ALS. The cause of the non-genetic forms of ALS is not known. Recent research from my laboratory and others in Tel Aviv, Hong Kong, and Atlanta suggest that the gut bacteria are involved in initiating the disease.

Conclusion

There are many causes of dementia. Every person with a complaint of significant memory impairment needs a comprehensive examination by a person experienced and interested in the area. The brain in aging is sensitive to changes in the internal and external environment, involving all organ systems. This suggests that attention to lifestyle factors, involving the four reserve factors, will assist in slowing progression and delaying onset. Attention to systemic health can lower the risk of dementing disorders and improve cognitive function with age.

Attention to systemic health can lower the risk of dementing disorders and improve cognitive function with age.

I am sorry to say that if everything is clear to you now, you haven't been paying attention. We don't know which molecules are most responsible for declining function in the brain and other structures in aging-related diseases. And we don't know what is responsible for the effects of aging on the brain in the absence of disease. What is the cause of Alzheimer's disease, Parkinson's disease, or ALS in cases that are not inherited (90–99 percent of the cases)? Is inflammation the trigger of neurodegeneration, or is neurodegeneration the trigger of inflammation? What is the role of the deposition of misfolded proteins? These matters have been vigorously debated in scientific circles for many years. While these important questions remain, we can learn from current research that there are things that we can all do to lower our risk through enhancement of our four multiple reserves factors.

There are remarkable similarities between the three main neurodegenerative diseases: Alzheimer's, Parkinson's, and ALS:

- they are usually not caused by genes;
- they have uncommon genetic forms which are autosomal dominant (they affect men and women equally and only one copy of the defective gene is needed for disease);
- they are associated with deposition in the brain of abnormally folded protein aggregates with toxic properties;

- they all have aging as the main risk factors;
- they are all associated with neuronal loss and loss of synapses;
- they all have a developmental pathway which is compatible with a spreading of a pathogenic (disease) process from one area of the body to another;
- they all have prominent features of excessive inflammation and free radicals in the brain;
- they all have slow onset including a 1–2 decade time when the disease is developing before the onset of signs or symptoms; and
- the risk of all of these conditions may be influenced by attention to the four factors, and lifelong enhancement through our actions on our cognitive, physical, psychological, and social reserves.

These commonalities are exciting because they suggest that a breakthrough in one area may lead to effective therapies for more than one condition.

There is a powerful tendency to reduce complexities into easier to understand concepts. Although this is largely unavoidable, we must always be aware of this process of simplification so we will not be deluded into believing that our understanding is deeper than it really is. We can appreciate the wisdom of Albert Einstein, who is often quoted as having said, "Everything should be made as simple as possible, but no simpler." However, what he actually said was "It can scarcely be denied that the supreme goal of all theory is to make the irreducible basic elements as simple and as few as possible without having to surrender the adequate representation of a single datum of experience."[70] Perhaps he is warning us not to lose sight of the forest for the trees, and also not to lose sight of the trees for the forest.

6 STROKE AND VASCULAR COGNITIVE IMPAIRMENT

Thoroughly conscious ignorance is the prelude to every real advance in science.
James Clerk Maxwell (1831–1897), Scottish mathematician, and scientist responsible for the classical theory of electromagnetic radiation

Many years ago, I attended a neurology conference and heard a distinguished physician give a talk about stroke. The doctor had received an award and was speaking to a room of several thousand people. His speech came after another physician had spoken about Alzheimer's disease.

The doctor who'd received the award began his speech by saying that he was glad his work focused on strokes, because unlike Alzheimer's disease, the causes of strokes are known.

I found this statement perplexing and wrote him a brief email congratulating him for his award, then asked him what he meant by saying that the causes of strokes were known. He responded by writing that strokes are caused by thromboses, hemorrhages, and embolisms. A thrombosis is when a blood vessel becomes blocked because of the accumulation of platelets and white blood cells. A hemorrhage is the leaking of a blood vessel and an embolism is when a clot moves from one part of the circulation to another, such as from the heart to the brain.

I found this physician's response disturbing. Thromboses, hemorrhages, and embolisms are not the *causes* of stroke, they are some of the *mechanisms* of stroke. It is important we realize that we often don't know what is causing a person to have a thrombosis, hemorrhage, or an embolism in the brain. As you will see, we know the risk factors for stroke, but risk factors are *not* causes.

What Are Cerebrovascular Diseases?

Vascular (blood vessel) factors are important for brain health and fitness throughout life. Cerebrovascular disease involves the large, middle, and small vessels of the neck and the brain. Abnormal growth of fibrous tissue (with fibers) and the deposition of platelets, immune blood cells, and lipids on the inside lining in the brain's blood vessels can cause narrowing. This narrowing of vessels impairs the opportunity for blood to flow and causes damage to the brain. An area of the brain which has been damaged by a lack of blood flow is called an infarct. It can be large, small, or microscopic (a microinfarct) and can damage cognitive function. Also, disease in the small vessels of the brain can diminish cognitive reserve and contribute to the development of both Alzheimer's and Parkinson's diseases, as well as increasing the chance that those people, in the early stages of the diseases already, will have impaired function.[21,71]

The vessel-narrowing process involves binding of platelets and lipids to the lining of large and small arteries and the formation of plaques (lipid deposits), which may be from the clotting of cellular elements. Vessel narrowing can also be due to thickening of the vessel wall. These processes impair clearance from the brain of important molecules, such as amyloid beta, which are involved in neuronal death, associated with Alzheimer's disease. Atherosclerosis is the process of vessel degeneration, previously called hardening of the arteries, in which the ability of the vessel to deliver blood is decreased. Atherosclerosis is often associated with lipid deposits, and it is now clear that the disease process also involves abnormal activation of the immune system. Vessel changes with age are highly linked to both activities and diet. Exercising multiple times per week and eating a high-fiber, vegetable-rich diet are good for you at all ages, and absolutely necessary as one ages. Without these activities, people risk dying young or suffering from dementia.

Strokes are the second leading cause of death in the world and the major cause of disability.

Strokes are the second leading cause of death in the world and the major cause of disability. Brain imaging has revealed that over 20 percent of people over the age of 65 have evidence of a small stroke that caused no clear symptoms. Strokes are often acute, with rapid onset and progression of symptoms. The brain can also be damaged by a long-term lack of sufficient blood flow, with loss of the axons which allow neurons to communicate with each other.

Why Is the Brain So Sensitive to Injury?

The brain is the most metabolically intense part of the body (as discussed in Chapter 3). This is because the work of the brain involves a continuity of electrical activity during wakefulness and sleep. Also, the brain has severely limited stores of oxygen and glucose, which must be continuously supplied. Neuronal activity inside the brain can only be maintained for 30–60 seconds without this continuous support. The brain uses glucose as its main energy source and will quickly stop working if glucose is not constantly supplied. All of the other tissues in the body have other potential sources of energy, but the brain's choices are limited. Because of these demands the brain has been equipped with an excellent support system of

blood vessels, which can meet the great metabolic requirements of our continuously active neurons. The vessels in
the neck and at the base of the brain have alternative pathways, called collaterals, so that if there is a problem with
one vessel, its work may be carried out by another. However, once the vessels leave the neck and the base of the
brain there are only poor alternative pathways available,
and blockage can cause significant damage.

What Happens during a Stroke?

This is what develops when a stroke occurs: the supply of
oxygen and glucose to the brain is not able to meet the
metabolic demand of the tissue and neurons, and other
cells die. This may be because of a clot in the blood vessel, called a thrombosis. It may also be because the clot
has traveled from somewhere else and lodged in a brain
vessel (embolism). A stroke may also be caused by bleeding into the brain or onto the external surface of the brain
(hemorrhage). Strokes may also be caused by a lack of sufficient supply of glucose and oxygen in the blood (without a thrombosis, embolism, or hemorrhage) because of
dehydration, bleeding, heart failure, low heart rate, low
blood sugar, low blood oxygen level, anemia (low red cell
count in the blood), and other causes. Thus, an infarct can
be caused by any of these four mechanisms: thrombosis,
embolism, hemorrhage, or insufficiency.

Vascular damage to the brain can cause sudden onset of
localized symptoms, such as weakness on one side with or
without sensory deficit. There may also be slow onset of
mild cognitive impairment or dementia. In the past, dementia of vascular origin was referred to incorrectly as "a
hardening of the arteries in the neck." It is now known
that dementia caused by vascular changes is not often
caused by narrowing of the blood vessels in the neck that

supply the brain. Dementia caused by a problem with the brain's circulation was also previously called multi-infarct dementia, or vascular dementia. The current term vascular cognitive impairment encompasses both dementia and mild cognitive impairment as a consequence of vascular damage to the brain, not only strokes. Vascular cognitive impairment includes several mechanisms including large, small, and microscopic strokes, large and small hemorrhages, damage from poor vascular regulation, white matter degeneration caused by small brain vessel disease, and vasculitis (inflammation in blood vessels). White matter changes in the brain caused by vascular disease can also be caused by loss of the neurons that are the cells of origin of the white matter fibers. Risk factors for vascular cognitive impairment are the same as the risk factors for stroke.[72,73]

Stroke Risk Factors

The main risk factors for a stroke are age, hypertension, smoking, diabetes, alcoholism, obesity, high-fat diet, high blood lipids, lack of physical activity, atrial fibrillation, cardiovascular disease, poor oral hygiene, periodontitis (an oral bacterial infection), a previous stroke, and a history of stroke in the family. Genes are also involved in stroke risk. However, Case Study 6 demonstrates the importance of interdependent interactions among the multiple reserve factors.

The risk factors for stroke illustrate the importance of interactions of the internal environment with the brain.

The risk factors for stroke illustrate the importance of interactions of the internal environment with the brain. Hypertension damages blood vessels throughout the body, including the brain, and contributes to small and large strokes. Diabetes also damages small blood vessels throughout the body, including the brain, and can contribute to large and small infarcts. In the United States, strokes are more common in African Americans than non-Hispanic white people, most likely related to a higher prevalence of hypertension.[61] The stroke risk is higher in people who gain weight in early adult life and have less physical activity. People who exercise vigorously not only have fewer strokes and less cognitive impairment resulting from strokes, they also have fewer complications, less severe strokes, and less of a risk of dying from a stroke.

Case Study 6

A thought experiment can help understand the role of genetic and environmental factors and disease. Consider this scenario: A 73-year-old man with hypertension (high blood pressure), who has smoked two packs of cigarettes per day for many years, was physically inactive and had progressive memory loss over three years, was found to have dementia of moderate severity. A neurological examination and blood tests did not suggest any cause for his dementia. MRI showed severe damage to the white matter throughout his brain, which impairs the ability of the cortex to communicate with itself and the rest of the brain. There were also small infarcts near the center of the brain, called lacunes (little lakes). It is highly likely that this problem is of vascular origin, referred to as vascular cognitive impairment. It is correct to say this condition is likely related to his age, smoking, physical inactivity, and hypertension.

But would we be surprised if we were told that his 78-year-old older brother also had hypertension, was more physically inactive and smoked more, but did not have this problem? No, we would not be surprised.

Thus, we cannot say that this person's illness was caused by age, smoking, and hypertension if his brother had all those features and was not affected. The difference between the two brothers may be linked to genetics, diet, obesity, and the microbiome. The critical factor causing his dementia is the interdependent interactions among his multiple reserve factors. His physical reserve is dependent upon his activities, genes, toxic exposures (smoking), and diet. His cognitive reserve is defined by his mental activities and the development of resilient networks in the brain. His psychological and social reserves are related to his ability to respond well to stress and maintain a healthy level of participation in the world.

There is a lot about these interactions that we do not know. Awareness of this ignorance is important for future advances. It is only now that the important role of the gut bacteria in cerebrovascular disease is beginning to be addressed. Stroke and vascular cognitive impairment are influenced by all four reserve factors: cognitive reserve may determine the effect a small stroke has on behavior (a person with a high reserve factor may be less affected than one with a low factor). High physical reserve will help to limit hypertension, diabetes, and obesity (all stroke risk factors). Physical reserve incudes the maintenance of normal blood pressure and kidney function, which are also linked to hypertension. Psychological and social reserves are important for the avoidance of depression, the maintenance of physical activity, and the avoidance of frailty.

In the words of the Italian astronomer Galileo Galilei (1564–1642): "To be human, we must ever be ready to pronounce that wise, ingenious and model statement, 'I do not know'."

Stroke and Alzheimer's Disease

With aging, vascular changes often occur together with neurodegenerative disorders, particularly Alzheimer's disease. The presence of small or large strokes increases the likelihood that a diagnosis of Alzheimer's disease will be made. This is probably because the damage to the brain caused by a stroke diminishes the cognitive reserve, so that a certain amount of Alzheimer's pathology in the brain will be more likely to cause impairment. It is also believed that vascular changes accelerate the Alzheimer's process directly. Furthermore, the deposition of the Alzheimer's-related protein amyloid beta in small brain vessels may lead to vascular damage to neurons and their pathways, and to small and large hemorrhages (referred to as cerebral amyloid angiopathy). Risk factors for vascular disease are also highly linked to Alzheimer's disease (particularly hypertension, obesity, physical inactivity, periodontitis, and diabetes).

Stroke and the Microbiota

Although we know the risk factors for stroke, we do not understand why many persons are affected. There is substantial evidence that the microbiota are involved.[73,74] Bacteria normally found in the mouth have been seen in abnormal blood vessels in people with strokes. Persons with periodontitis, the most common bacterial infection in the mouth, have a higher risk of stroke, as well as hypertension, heart disease, and Alzheimer's disease, compared to those without periodontitis. Workers at the Cleveland Clinic in Cleveland, Ohio, led by Dr. Stanley Hazen, have shown that gut bacteria metabolize compounds from meat, cheese, and eggs to create a molecule (trimethylamine) which, when oxidized by the liver, can travel in the blood, and accelerate the vessel-narrowing process responsible for cardiovascular disease and stroke.[75] Also, with colleagues in Japan, my group has shown that oral bacteria can travel in the blood to brain vessels and contribute to small and large hemorrhages.[73,74] We have also proposed that bacteria in the gut and mouth can accelerate aggregation (clumping) of proteins that occurs in blood vessels in Alzheimer's disease.[56]

Cerebrovascular disease makes a very important contribution to cognitive impairment with aging. It is critical to recognize that lifestyle factors play a large role in the risk of all forms of stroke.

Cerebrovascular disease makes a very important contribution to cognitive impairment with aging. It is critical to recognize that lifestyle factors play a large role in the risk of all forms of stroke. Important is the fact that no one can assess their risk of stroke by how they feel. Atrial fibrillation is a common abnormality of the heart rhythm, which may have no symptoms. In this condition, the left atrium does not fully empty, and blood clots may develop, which can be transmitted to the brain to cause small or late strokes. Similarly, hypertension, the most important risk factor for stroke, usually causes no symptoms whatsoever.

Stroke Warning Signs

Everyone should know the warning signs for an acute stroke, because there are now powerful tools and procedures that may reverse the vascular damage, if recognized soon enough (time is critical for recovery). Remember the American Heart Association's BE FAST mnemonic device for remembering the warning signs of stroke: Balance, Eyes, Face, Arm, Speech, Time. These warning signs include: sudden numbness; weakness in face, arm, or leg, especially only one side of the body; difficulty seeing; trouble walking; and a severe headache.

What Can We Do to Lessen Stroke Risk?

In order to control the risk of stroke and vascular cognitive impairment it is important to manage hypertension, exercise frequently, avoid alcohol abuse and smoking, practice good oral hygiene, avoid obesity, and avoid a high-salt, high-fat (particularly saturated fat), low-fiber diet. The lifestyle measures reviewed in Part II of the book, Chapters 12–25, will also lower the risk of having a stroke.

7 OTHER DEMENTIAS

Although Alzheimer's disease is the most common cause of dementia, it isn't the only cause. If you or a loved one is experiencing memory loss, it's important to get a proper diagnosis as soon as possible.

As many as 10–20 percent of people with dementia may have a treatable or reversible disorder. That's a sign of optimism.

As many as 10–20 percent of people with dementia may have a treatable or reversible disorder. That's a sign of optimism.

Normal Pressure Hydrocephalus

An uncommon condition called normal pressure hydrocephalus (NPH) is particularly critical to recognize because it is a potentially reversible cause of dementia. NPH is characterized by obstruction of the outflow of cerebrospinal fluid (CSF) in the brain and causes gait disturbance, difficulty with urination, and cognitive deficits. The gait disturbance is often highly characteristic, as it has been referred to as magnetic, in that the person walks as if his or her feet are magnetized to the floor and are difficult to lift. In NPH, this problem is not caused by weakness. If there is a characteristic pattern on the MRI of the brain, a high-volume spinal tap or CSF drainage procedure may help with the diagnosis. The surgical placement of a shunt to provide an alternate pathway for CSF absorption may be curative.

Creutzfeldt–Jakob Disease and Bovine Spongiform Encephalopathy

Another rare disorder is Creutzfeldt–Jakob disease (CJD), which is a rapidly progressive dementia that advances from first symptoms to death, usually in less than one year (see Case Study 7). It may be caused by mutations in a gene called the prion protein, the function of which has not yet been established. However, in both genetic and non-genetic cases, an abnormally configured shape of the protein develops. This abnormal shape is transmissible and can cause an abnormal configuration of other molecules of the same protein.

The concept of the prion disorders began with the discovery of scrapie, a fatal, degenerative disease found in sheep. The name scrapie was derived from the fact that the sheep scraped off their fur because of a neuronal degeneration. The disease was found over 250 years ago to be transmissible from animal to animal. In the 1950s, an epidemic of a brain degeneration, called kuru, was observed in Eastern New Guinea. The US National Institutes of Health sent Daniel Carleton Gajdusek, a pediatrician scientist, to research the disorder. He lived for years in the highlands of New Guinea, learned all the local languages, and carried out extensive investigations. He found no evidence of a toxic, nutritional, genetic, metabolic, traumatic, or infectious origin of the malady. Notably, there was no evidence in the brain of an infectious process.

The nature of the illness remained unclear until the British veterinary pathologist William Hadlow wrote to Gajdusek in 1959 to remark that the pathology of kuru in the brain was highly similar to that of scrapie. Because of this observation, Gajdusek and collaborators inoculated brain material from affected persons into the brains of chimpanzees. After several years, the animals developed the disease. This led to a remarkable series of studies showing that the infectious agent in kuru, as well as CJD, is an abnormally formed protein that lacks nucleic acids. (Gadjusek and colleagues acknowledged the contributions of chimpanzees Daisey, Joanne, and Georgette to the research in their 1966 paper, which was published in the journal *Nature*.[76]) The prion concept was developed through an important series of elegant studies by Stanley Prusiner. Both Gadjusek and Prusiner received Nobel Prizes in Physiology or Medicine for their contributions.

In the 1980s, an epidemic brain degeneration was found in cattle in the United Kingdom. The pathology of the disorder was highly similar to that of scrapie, kuru, and CJD. Despite this similarity of the two conditions, the danger of eating infected cattle was initially dismissed by the British government. It was originally thought that scrapie could not be transmitted from sheep to cattle. It was later believed that the condition, called bovine spongiform encephalopathy (BSE or mad cow disease), could not be transmitted from cattle to humans. All of these original beliefs were wrong. The epidemic in cows has been linked to the process of feeding rendered material from cows to other cows.[1] More than 225 people died after eating infected beef and contracting BSE. CJD and BSE are both untreatable currently.

---

[1] At the time the crisis of BSE was developing in the United Kingdom, the Agriculture Minister, John Gummer, fed a burger to his four-year-old daughter at a press conference to show how safe it was. Unfortunately, he was mistaken. A video of the event is available here: www.youtube.com/watch?v=QobuvWX_Grc.

Stanley Prusiner and many others worldwide are working on developing a therapy. The concept of the prion disorders is based upon the transmissibility of an abnormally configured protein structure. It is now believed that similar processes are involved in Alzheimer's disease, Parkinson's disease, and amyotrophic lateral sclerosis (see Chapter 5). Contrary to the findings for BSE, there is no evidence that these diseases are transmitted between persons or from animals to humans.

Nowadays, the risk of BSE has decreased because the process of feeding material from cows to cows has been banned globally. However, fish raised on fish farms may be fed material from cows, and fish are able to be infected with the prion. In my opinion, ground-up cow carcasses should not be fed to fish. It seems to me that fish do perfectly well in the sea without eating cows. The problem, of course, is economical – renderers need to find a buyer for their product. (Rendering is the conversion of animal tissue into stable, usable materials.)

Along with several co-authors, I published a paper in 2009 suggesting that cows should not be fed to fish because of the risk of infection of the fish with a BSE agent. Also, fish can be a carrier of the agent, which is highly resistant to inactivation.[77] Following publication, the director of a renderers' association called me with concern. He asked, "What can we do with unwanted items from the slaughter of cows if they can't be used in fish farming?" I suggested that they be burnt (he wasn't happy with my suggestion). An additional concern is that the nutritional value of fish is related to the diet of the fish. Fish who eat beef may not have the same levels of omega-3 polyunsaturated fatty acids that are beneficial to humans as fish eating their normal diet. Also of concern is the fact that BSE can develop spontaneously in cows; it is not necessary for the cow to have received an infectious agent from another cow. Just as CJD can spontaneously develop in a human

Case Study 7
A 42-year-old male patient of mine had a five-month history of rapidly progressive dementia with violent outbursts, hitting his wife, and waking up in the middle of the night. An electroencephalogram was highly abnormal with epileptic activity. There was no report of neurological or psychiatric disease in his family. He was moderately demented and could not name the previous president. He developed difficulty with visual perception and walked into objects. When he walked toward a window with venetian blinds, he thought it was a staircase. In tests, the CSF showed signs of CJD and MRI showed extensive asymmetric changes in the cerebral cortex typical for the disease. After six months of rapid progression, the patient died of CJD.

without a genetic anomaly or exposure to prions, BSE can spontaneously develop in a cow. In the European Union and Japan, most animals are tested for BSE. In the United States, animals are not routinely tested for BSE.

Chronic Traumatic Encephalopathy

Scientific advances have demonstrated that playing American football is associated with a high risk of an incurable neurodegenerative disease called chronic traumatic encephalopathy (CTE).[78] The National Football League (NFL) has recognized the harmful influences of the game on brain function, as indicated by its $765 million concussion settlement with former players. Today, there is ample information available to show that head injuries are bad for the brain: big injuries are bad and little injuries are bad, especially when they are repetitive. Perhaps the greatest wisdom comes from Hippocrates, who said, "No head injury is too severe to despair of, nor too trivial to ignore."

Today, there is ample information available to show that head injuries are bad for the brain: big injuries are bad and little injuries are bad, especially when they are repetitive.

The risk of the development of CTE has been well documented in both college and professional American football players. We know now that multiple mild, moderate, or severe head injuries cause damage to the brain that can lead to this chronic, progressive, and untreatable disorder. Subjects with CTE are found to have progressive degeneration in the frontal lobes, amygdala, hippocampus, and medial temporal lobes of the brain, and demonstrate cognitive deterioration, loss of motor abilities, agitation, depression, and suicidal thoughts. The neuropathology of CTE has been found to be positively correlated with years of playing the high-impact sport, where hits are celebrated (the risk is higher, the longer people play). CTE can only be diagnosed after death. In a recent study of 202 former National Football League football players, CTE was found in 87 percent of the players' brains.

The reason that society has not widely recognized the profound influence of head injuries in football is because the effects are both hidden and delayed. We see many occasions where blows to the head are received, in every game of American football. When the player's performance is affected (he has had his "bell rung"), the change is usually brief. These events often have little or no visible effect on the player at that moment. However, the belief that these shocks have no lasting effect on the brain is clearly an illusion.

Consider the woodpecker, which was one of the first examples of adaptive evolution revealed by Charles

Darwin, and whose "feet, tail, beak and tongue" are "admirably adapted to catch insects under the bark of trees."[79] The woodpecker drums its head against a tree at a speed of more than 20 times per second. It is only able to endure the forces sustained while feeding because its head, beak, and tongue have been adapted through natural selection to protect the brain from the repetitive forces of smashing its beak into trees. This mechanism has allowed woodpeckers to use their heads for food gathering in an effective and safe way for many millions of years. But evolution has not come up with a good mechanism through which the human brain can be protected from forces applied to the head, such as occurs in football. The brain damage football players suffer is not visible. We are deluded by the remarkable ability of the brain to maintain or regain consciousness after blows to the head. However, this recovery masks the initiation of brain pathology.

Tragically, there is no valid diagnostic test at the moment for CTE and no effective treatment. It is painfully obvious that people should not participate in a sport with a high risk of head injury. These sorts of sports are especially hazardous for children, as their brains are not fully developed until the end of the second decade of life, and thus they are more vulnerable to physical damage. Injuries to the head sustained in early life through sporting activities may also cause problems later, because of lower cognitive reserve.

Other Conditions

There are also several other uncommon neurodegenerative diseases. These include progressive supranuclear palsy, characterized by features of Parkinson's disease (referred to as parkinsonism), difficulty with up and down eye movements, dizziness, vertigo, falling, and unsteadiness. Multiple system atrophy is a non-genetic condition in which there are also features of Parkinson's disease, including poor balance and coordination, bladder problems, cognitive difficulties, and poor control of blood pressure. In cortical basal degeneration there may also be parkinsonism with stiffness, dementia, weakness, and asymmetrical motor abnormalities.

A wide range of systemic problems that are not primarily neurological may also cause dementia. These conditions may primarily affect every one of the body's organ systems. The commonest cause of dementia in Germany in 1907, when Alois Alzheimer reported his first case of early-onset dementia, was syphilis of the nervous system. The commonest cause of dementia in people under 50 years of age today in New York City is HIV/AIDS.

Alcohol and the Brain

Alcohol abuse is a common cause of dementia. There are several ways in which excessive alcohol intake can damage the brain. First of all, ethanol is directly toxic to neurons. With age, the ability of the liver to detoxify alcohol and lower blood alcohol levels is impaired. Thus, persons who drink three drinks a day may begin to have cognitive problems into their 80s because of their aged liver's diminished ability to metabolize alcohol. Second, people who drink too much are often nutritionally deprived and can have a relatively sudden onset of dementia with psychosis caused by thiamine deficiency (vitamin B1) (this is called the Wernicke Korsakoff syndrome). There may also be malnutrition for other nutrients in alcoholic persons, other than thiamine. Alcohol abuse is also associated with epilepsy and head injuries from falling. Alcoholic persons may develop liver damage which can severely impair the function of the central nervous system. Remarkably, subjects with cognitive impairment caused by alcohol abuse may recover partially or completely if they are able to be continuously abstinent for a prolonged period of time. Scientific studies have shown a recovery of lost brain structures in alcoholic people who stop drinking.

Remarkably, subjects with cognitive impairment caused by alcohol abuse may recover partially or completely if they are able to be continuously abstinent for a prolonged period of time.

Conclusions

A wide range of conditions may cause dementia other than Alzheimer's disease. A comprehensive evaluation must be performed in each case. Also, our ability to appreciate the opportunity of aging is related to the functional capacities of our four reserve factors, which requires us to avoid head injury and excess alcohol consumption.

8 OUR MICROBIOTA AND HOW TO DO GENE THERAPY IN THE KITCHEN

Without symbiosis, life on Earth as we see it today would not exist.

Eran Elinav, Israeli microbiota researcher[80]

Introduction to the Microbiota

Our bodies are home to a vast sea of microorganisms. They reside inside us and on all our body surfaces. There are as many cells of these microbial – microscopic – partners as there are our own cells. The word microbiota describes all the organisms that are living with us.

The important role of these partners of ours in our health and fitness has only been realized in the past 10 years. They are invisible and do not receive the attention they deserve. The microbiota are a key component of our physical reserve. I know that this is a strange and new concept to many. Before I outline the nature of these communities, I will share this story in order to illustrate a critical point of the book – that the gut bacteria are vital to our health and fitness.

Human breast milk contains complex sugars, referred to as oligosaccharides, that cannot be digested by the baby. There are more of these molecules in human breast milk than protein. There are over 200 different structures of these molecules.[81] When I read about this I was astounded. How is that possible? Why would evolution produce these complex sugars that can't be used by the baby? The answer: babies are born without a well-developed bacterial community in the gut. While the baby can't digest these sugars, they feed gut bacteria, which must establish a stable population inside the baby to encourage the health and development of the baby's brain and immune system.

This is a powerful illustration of the importance of the bacteria for our well-being. The good news is that there are many things we can all do to improve our bacterial partners, which can enhance our aging. There is a paradox concerning our microbiota: we are not aware of them, yet they live on us and in us, and we can detect products of their fermentation. We deal with them every day through our dietary choices, without an awareness of the role they play in our lives. The microbiota are a central hub of our control systems, and are critical for health. The nature of the microbial communities we harbor are under our control. Our actions influence our partner organisms and impact their role in our health and fitness.

The nature of the microbial communities we harbor are under our control. Our actions influence our partner organisms and impact their role in our health and fitness.

Our partner microbes are collectively referred to as the microbiota, and their genes and the genetic information they contain is called the metagenome or the microbiome. They should not be called "flora" or "microflora," as they are not plants. Their communities are comprised of bacteria, viruses, fungi, protozoa, parasites, and other microbial organisms. They are with us from birth throughout life, and have evolved with us. Even a billion years ago, our ancestors all had microbiota.

The Location and Nature of Our Microbes

There are trillions and trillions of microbes (mostly viruses and bacteria) in and on our bodies. We also have twice as many viruses as bacteria inside us. Most of the viruses in the gut only infect bacteria, and do not damage humans. Our microbiota reside on the skin, in sweat glands, hair follicles, eyes, ears, nose, mouth, pharynx, larynx, and all parts of our intestine. Most of them have been identified only because of new genetic techniques that allow scientists to study their genes (sequencing of their DNA allows for precise identification and analysis). Astoundingly, our bodies possess one hundred times more microbial genetic information than human genetic information.

Many of the microbial partners that inhabit us are symbionts or mutualists. This kind of relationship is one where both partners benefit. For example, non-pathogenic skin bacteria help to prevent dangerous bacteria from gaining a foothold. We help these organisms by providing a place for them to live and harvest valuable nutrients. Symbiotic relationships are critical to biology.[1]

Our microbiota are part of who we are. We cannot remove them and if we could it would be a really bad idea. The surface area of the gastrointestinal tract is about three-quarters of the area of a tennis court, and this is where the microbiota influence our health and disease. About 10 percent of the substances we ingest and used by the body to provide energy are of bacterial origin.

Why Are the Microbiota Important?

Microbiota influence all of our organ systems, assist in digestion, disease resistance, contribute to metabolism, and are critical for the maintenance of health and fitness.

[1]   Symbiosis is when two different organisms live together, benefiting both.

A key step in uncovering the influence of the microbiota came with studies of germ-free animals. These are animals (usually mice) that have been raised in an environment free of microbes. Surprisingly, this work showed how an absence of microbes resulted in abnormalities of immunity, metabolism, and behavior. Germ-free mice have defective immune systems. It appears that exposure to gut bacteria is needed to educate the immune system on how to develop. The wide range of influences of the microbiota are shown in Tables 3 and 4.

Table 3 *Diseases and processes influenced by the microbiota*

Anxiety	Harvesting of nutrition from the gut
Asthma	Immunity
Autism	Inflammatory bowel disease
Allergies	Learning and memory
Blood–brain barrier	Liver disease
permeability	Metabolism
Brain development	Microglia function
Cancer	Multiple sclerosis
Cardiovascular disease	Neurodegenerative disorders
Cerebrovascular disease	(Alzheimer's disease, Parkinson's
Circadian clock	disease, ALS)
Diabetes (insulin	Obesity
responsiveness)	Production of vitamins and
Depression	essential amino acids (K, B3, folate)
Digestion of nutrients	Resistance from pathogens
Drug metabolism and	(disease-causing agents)
degradation of environmental	Resistance to famine
chemicals	Satiety (feeling that one has eaten
Fat storage	enough)
Gut–blood barrier permeability	Sociability
	Stress responses
	Stroke

Table 4 *Examples of the influence of the microbiota on the body*

- Bacteria in the nose can stimulate small molecules that inhibit the growth of other potentially harmful bacteria.[82]
- Dietary intake of salt can increase inflammation in the body, through actions on the microbiota and possibly increase the Alzheimer's process in the brain.[83]
- Transfer of organisms from obese animals to animals lacking bacteria causes weight gain in the recipient animals. Obesity may be associated with an enhanced ability of the gut bacteria to obtain energy from the diet (harvesting), so that modulation of the microbiota may be a new approach to obesity.
- Metabolic products of the microbiota influence satiety, the perception leading to the cessation of feeding.
- Microbiota in the skin enhance wound healing.
- The gut microbiota of pregnant mice influence the immune and central nervous system functions of babies, including the development of autism, obesity, and diabetes.[84]
- The microbiota affect the way proteins are made by changing the packaging of DNA and, in doing so, regulate inflammation.[85]
- Bacteria have metabolic products that are bioactive metabolites, which can influence neuronal transmission and growth of neurons and synapses, as well as myelination (development of insulation on axons) and behavior.
- The influence of smoking, obesity, and alcohol on cardiovascular disease may operate through the microbiota.[86]
- Diets lacking fiber my cause erosion of the mucus layer of the intestine, leading to inflammation in the body and accelerating DNA damage that promotes tumor formation.[87]
- Gut bacteria can protect against heavy-metal toxicity.
- Dysbiosis is related to depression, anxiety, and cognitive impairment.

Table 4 *(cont.)*

- Dysbiosis can be caused by agricultural chemicals and artificial sweeteners.
- Gut bacteria influence insulin resistance and diabetes.
- Microbiota metabolize foreign molecules including toxins and drugs, perhaps as much as the liver, and may protect us from toxins (they may also produce toxins from environmental molecules).
- Gut bacteria contribute to cancer creation, dissemination, and prevention.
- Gut bacteria keep the intestinal barrier strong and help to keep environment proteins and pathogens out.
- The microbiota can diminish the toxicity of therapeutic radiation.

Colonization versus Infection

It's critical to understand that the presence of these bacteria in our bodies isn't an infection.

It's critical to understand that the presence of these bacteria in our bodies isn't an infection. When microbes grow in an abnormal manner, in a place where they don't belong and cause disease, that's an infection. Our microbiota are present at all times and help to prevent infection by stably occupying a place in or on our bodies that makes it difficult for harmful organisms to flourish. This is referred to as colonization, not infection, and provides our bodies with "home field advantage" to stave off intruders that may harm us. When the population of bacteria are not supportive of health, a state of dysbiosis is observed (e.g., lower diversity of organisms). The interaction of our body and the microbiota go both ways: it has been said that the immune system "gardens" the microbiota and chooses which organisms can become residents.

Infectious agents have been associated with neurode-generative disease for many years. Viruses can remain dormant in the nervous system after infection for decades. Several researchers have shown evidence that herpes viruses may remain latent and participate in causing Alzheimer's disease. Some scientists have suggested that this disease is initiated by the reactivation of herpes simplex 1 and 2 or human herpes virus 6 in the brain, which were acquired during childhood. Reactivation of these viruses may be related to enhanced brain inflammation caused by peripheral infections.[88] The best example of a disease caused by a latent virus is shingles, which is caused by the varicella zoster virus (also called herpes zoster) that triggers a mild illness in children called chickenpox. The virus often becomes resident in the body, with the risk of reactivation as shingles, causing skin eruption and pain many decades later. This is also an excellent example of the importance of our physical reserve factor, as the risk of shingles reactivation in older people is related to the presence of cancer, immunosuppressive medications, steroids, vitamin D deficiency, diabetes, and systemic illness. Critically, people over 50 years of age can be protected from shingles infection with a vaccine. Unfortunately, vaccine approaches to the treatment of Alzheimer's disease based on development of an immune response to the amyloid-beta protein haven't been shown to be effective. However, an awareness of the microbiota and the need for dietary diversity may be of preventive value, as our microbiota are a critical component of our physical reserve.

Diversity and the Microbiota

A critical feature of the microbiota is their diversity – a wide variety of organisms are present. The greatest concentration of bacteria in our bodies is found in the colon, and adults have perhaps one to two kilograms of living bacteria in the gut at all times. Studies of hunter–gatherer populations living today suggest that our ancestors had an even wider range of microbiota than we have now, because of their more varied diet. This is excellent support for the need for all of us to have a highly diverse diet. During my one-year sabbatical leave in Japan, I noted that a lunch may involve over 20 different items, whereas a cheese sandwich may have only two or three. Diversity in food feeds lots of different bacteria in the gut and it is good for health to have many kinds of microbes living there.

With aging, the normally great diversity of bacteria in the gut decreases due to a less varied diet. This decrease in diversity is correlated with age-related diseases, particularly frailty, which is a condition with greatly reduced reserve capacity. Because they have less diverse microbiota, the aged may have reduced resilience, so that the impact of antibiotics and illness may be more marked than otherwise. The reduced resilience of the microbiota with aging can be avoided with attention to dietary choices.

The Oral Microbiome

Although the majority of studies of the microbiota have focused on intestinal organisms, oral bacteria are also linked to brain and heart diseases. It is clear that our partner organisms in the mouth, throat, and sinuses also play critical roles in many processes important in human life.

Here's how it works: There are about 1,000 different species of microbes that live in the mouth, nose, and throat. A single milliliter of saliva may have as many as 100 million bacterial cells, which is pretty impressive when you think about it. Their presence makes it difficult for disease-causing organisms to grow (home field advantage, again). Many of the resident bacteria in the mouth can cause inflammation locally and systemically. The commonest kind of bacterial infection in the mouth is periodontitis, a gum infection that damages the attachment of teeth. Periodontitis is a risk factor for cardiovascular disease, as well as stroke and Alzheimer's disease. Scientists at the University of Louisville, led by Professor Jan Potempa, have found that an oral bacterium may infiltrate the brain and secrete toxins, which damage neurons.[89] A clinical trial of Alzheimer's using a small molecule which inhibits the bacteria's toxic effects is under way.

Studies have also shown that oral bacteria can influence the production of immune cells in the body to activate inflammation at many sites, including the brain. Such inflammatory influences can actively contribute to neurodegeneration. Research I'm involved in with colleagues in Osaka, Japan, has shown that oral bacteria also contribute to small and large strokes.[73] Oral health is a critical part of our physical reserve and attention to oral health helps to manage unhealthy microbiota in the mouth and throat (see Chapter 22).

Oral health is a critical part of our physical reserve and attention to oral health helps to manage unhealthy microbiota in the mouth and throat

---

We must understand the microbiota from an evolutionary perspective to appreciate their role in our physical reserve.

Co-evolution and the Microbiota

The wide-ranging influence of the gut bacteria can be understood by considering our evolution, as well as the evolution of bacteria. They play an important role in our health and avoidance of disease; therefore, it is necessary for the body to nurture the microbiota. In this scenario, we are the host, and the microbes are our partners.

Our history with the microbiota is best described by the word co-evolution. We evolved with them, and they evolved with us.

Our history with the microbiota is best described by the word co-evolution. We evolved with them, and they evolved with us. It is obviously necessary for the bacteria that our bodies tolerate their presence because we would mount a vigorous immunological attack if we considered them to be foreign invaders and pathogens (disease-causing organisms). If that happened, everyone would have inflammatory bowel disease or much, much worse. Our immune system has developed the capacity to recognize and monitor the contents of the microbiota and to tolerate their presence. The immune system removes unwanted organisms (weeds?), enhancing the growth of desirable ones.

Since diet influences the microbiota and diet varies around the world, are there influences of geography on bacterial populations?

The Microbiota and Disease around the World

A fascinating perspective on the microbiota is provided by considering global patterns of disease. Alzheimer's disease has been found to be less common in older people in India and Africa than in Europe and the United States. While working in Kenya on an Alzheimer's project, I met a former dean of the School of Medicine at the University of Nairobi. He was 76 years old and recounted how, when he was in medical school in the 1950s, a patient suffered a heart attack. Doctors and medical students visited him because they had never seen a person who had experienced such an ailment.

Our studies in rural Kenya showed people living there had an extremely low intake of saturated fat. This was especially true of Kenyans born in the mid-twentieth century. People told us that when they were young, they ate meat once or twice a year. This was because animals in their village were too precious for slaughter. Their diet consisted of corn, rice, beans, sweet potatoes, yams, and other vegetables and legumes. Did they use butter, chicken or beef fat, olive oil, margarine, or vegetable oil when cooking? Nope. Their plant products were cooked by boiling, the most low-fat option possible. The high level of plant consumption also provided high levels of dietary fiber.

The lower risk of Alzheimer's disease in Africans in comparison to many Americans may be due to Africans' higher consumption of fiber, as well a lower intake of saturated fat. Their higher level of physical activity, and greater physical reserve, may also be protective against the development of Alzheimer's disease (see Chapter 9). Africa is the most diverse continent on Earth and the situation in other areas of Africa may very well be different. Unfortunately, there has been relatively little research on age-related neurological disease in this continent.

Black Americans are at higher risk for Alzheimer's disease than Africans. The higher Alzheimer's disease risk in African Americans compared to Africans led us to develop a health literacy program in Cleveland, while I was working at the Case Western Reserve University. We partnered with African American churches to educate the public about the potentially modifiable risk factors for the disease. A special moment was when a pastor told his congregation that we should "be like Jesus, walk! Jesus didn't take the bus." The pastor encouraged the audience to eat the genuine "soul food," which was what their ancestors ate in Africa: beans, rice, legumes, vegetables, and not what is currently considered soul food: pork, ribs, fried chicken, macaroni and cheese. All of us, regardless of race, ethnicity, or religion, would benefit from the words of this wise pastor. Don't take the bus or drive your car to every destination: walk, jog, or bike. Or, if this isn't feasible, pick a parking spot a few blocks from work or walk to a bus stop one or two stops away. Every step matters on the road to a healthier life, and a plant-based high-fiber diet, low in meat, is best.

With support from the National Institute on Aging at the National Institutes of Health, I also studied Alzheimer's disease in the Middle East. My colleagues and I found that the disease was relatively more common in Arabs residing in Israel than in other countries. The factors responsible may include the relatively high occurrence in Arabs of a diet high in saturated fat, low levels of education, obesity, physical inactivity, hypertension, and low rates of fish consumption. We were surprised to find that the apolipoprotein E ε4 Alzheimer's disease risk gene was actually less common in Arabs than in other communities. This work was accomplished by Palestinian neurologists, who went door to door to evaluate older residents. A difficult problem they faced was that in every home they were greeted as a guest and expected to have a cup of Arabic coffee. I know from experience that it is not advisable to drink more than two or three cups of such coffee in the morning. But refusing the host's offer was impolite. (All in a day's work for science!)

How to Do "Gene Therapy in the Kitchen"

The good news about the microbiota is that it is relatively easy to change bacterial populations in the gut. Changing the bacterial DNA in the intestines can be done in as little as two weeks by altering diet. I call this "gene therapy in the kitchen." A good example of this is a remarkable study from Pittsburgh and South Africa. The risk of colon cancer is five to ten times more common in African Americans in the United States then in black Africans living in South Africa. Alzheimer's disease and cardiovascular disease are also less common in Africans compared to African Americans. The diet of many African Americans is higher in salt and saturated fat and lower in fiber than the diet of South Africans. This study changed the diet in the two communities, so that African Americans were consuming a diet similar to that of the South Africans and the South Africans were consuming an African American diet. After two weeks they found expected patterns of change in the microbiota, as well as changes in metabolism, so that the African Americans who were consuming a better diet had healthier microbiota, and the South Africans now had unhealthy microbiota. The changes demonstrated that the gut bacteria of the South Africans, who were now consuming the African American diet, provided their hosts with molecular signals indicating a higher risk of cancer and inflammatory diseases.[90]

The lesson here is that changes we make to our diet today can improve our health quickly. We all need to consider the opportunity to pursue gene therapy in the kitchen. Doing this is relatively straightforward: next time you dine at a restaurant, order the kale salad. When you're home, make a tofu stir fry instead of a pork stir fry. Skip the salty snack and reach for the apple instead. Better yet, don't buy the salty snack or ground hamburger or the chocolate ice cream with Oreos (really, you can do it!). Changing your diet is difficult, but not impossible (see Chapter 20).

I can't say enough about the importance of fiber in the diet. Eating fiber is critical to human health – and preventing Alzheimer's disease and dementia – yet few Americans eat enough brown rice, beans, nuts, berries, and other sources of fiber. Your body needs fiber because of the short-chain fatty acids (SCFAs) made by gut bacteria. These

SCFAs are small molecules that influence energy use in the body. The bacteria that make SCFAs love eating fiber as much as you love eating ice cream. Since SCFAs enhance gut bacterial health, their need for fiber is critical to your health. Studies show that people with Parkinson's disease and low levels of SCFAs are more likely to suffer cognitive impairment.

SCFAs help you to feel fuller for longer, to improve lipid levels, to better manage diabetes, and to enhance the health of the intestinal barrier, which prevents the potentially harmful contents of the intestine from entering the bloodstream. SCFAs also influence the way DNA is used in the immune system to produce more circulating immune cells, which serve to enhance tolerance by diminishing the aggression of immune responses. This is a generally beneficial effect, as aggressive immune responses (inflammation) are an important feature of several age-related diseases, including heart disease, diabetes, stroke, macular degeneration, cancer, and arthritis, as well as neurodegeneration. Dietary fiber has been found to have beneficial effects on cardiovascular disease, diabetes, and cancer. Less than 10 percent of Americans consume the recommended amount of dietary fiber.

The Microbiota and Immunity

There are several ways in which bacteria in the gut, including the mouth and nose, can influence our health. Their important influences on the immune system concern both inborn – or innate – responses (called the *innate immune system*) and the *adaptive immune system*. The innate immune system responds to potential threats very quickly, without the need for previous exposure. It has mechanisms to detect and rapidly respond to bacterial signals that it recognizes as hazardous and can recruit immune cells to sites of infection and activate immune responses with cells and immune molecules. The adaptive immune system allows for highly specific responses to be made depending upon previous exposures. For example, immunity to measles following vaccination is a response of the adaptive immune system. The functions of both the innate and adaptive immune systems are influenced by the microbiota.

Bacterial products may be beneficial for health, such as SCFAs. They may also be disease inducing. The molecule trimethylamine is made by gut bacteria and leads to more heart disease, stroke, and Alzheimer's disease. The bacteria that make this molcule are increased by meat and eggs in the diet. Functional bacterial amyloids are another bacterial product with negative effects on health.

Neurodegenerative Disease and the Microbiota

There have been limited advances in therapies for Alzheimer's disease and related disorders in the last 20 years. I believe that this is because most of the work in the area is devoted to showing *what* is going wrong. My approach is to ask *why* it is going wrong. The Nobel laureate Stanley Prusiner has suggested that the initiating factor in these brain diseases is the random development of an abnormal protein-folding structure. I find this explanation unsatisfying and prefer to consider the role that our largest environmental exposure (the microbiota) plays in age-related brain disease. Signals from the microbiota may serve to initiate disease processes in neurodegeneration.

Bacteria make molecules that are similar in their three-dimensional structure to the amyloid-beta protein found in Alzheimer's disease and the alpha synuclein protein found in Parkinson's disease. These microbial products are called functional bacterial amyloids because they help the bacteria to stick together, form communities, and resist destruction. Half of all bacteria make functional bacterial amyloids. (Amyloids are discussed in Chapter 5.)

In 2015, I proposed that bacterial amyloid proteins produced in the gut influence the misfolding of neuronal proteins.[56] Exposure to the amyloid structure of the bacteria can make proteins in neurons adopt a similar and disease-causing shape. We and others have shown that exposure to the bacterial amyloids prepares the immune system to make it more reactive to brain amyloid proteins. In all the neurodegenerative disorders, there are excessive immune reactions going on in the brain. This may be initiated by interactions of the immune system with bacteria in the gut. The immune system that has been exposed to bacterial amyloids is more ready for action, so that when it is exposed to neuronal amyloid, the immune reaction is more intense. These proposals have now been confirmed in our labs as well as by others in Israel, Hong Kong, Denmark, and Los Angeles.

These concepts concerning microbial influences on the brain are new for me and many others. In science, it is common to be devoted to a narrow area with intense focus. The fact that we have no effective disease-modifying treatments for the neurodegenerations suggests that a broader focus may help. The animal psychologist Wolfgang Kohler said:[91] "It would be interesting to inquire how many times essential advances in science have first been made by the fact that the boundaries of special disciplines were not respected ... Trespassing is one of the most successful techniques in science."

My research approach is best summarized by saying there is only one kind of science, and that is the study of everything with all available methods. I am pleased to be a trespasser.

It has been well established that many older people have considerable amyloid-beta protein deposits and neuritic plaques in the brain (both features of Alzheimer's disease) but are not cognitively impaired. It may be that as many as 50 percent of centenarians have significant pathology in the brain but aren't experiencing dementia. This may be because an immune response has not been directed against these age-related molecules.[56,92] Exposure to functional bacterial amyloid proteins made by the gut bacteria may enhance the reaction in the brain to the cerebral amyloids that normally develop with age. The microbiota have also been shown to influence the activity of the most important immune cells in the brain, the microglia.

Our microbiota are part of our physical reserve factor. This reveals an essential component of the concept of the reserves: the reserve factors influence disease processes and also influence the body's responses to these processes.

The reserve factors influence disease processes and also influence the body's responses to these processes.

The Gut–Brain Pathway

There are several avenues by which microbiota affect brain function and disease. Figure 5 shows routes with which microbes in the nose, mouth, and intestines may influence the brain and the spinal cord. Neuronal molecules (such as amyloid beta, tau, alpha-synuclein and others), microbial metabolic products as well as microbes themselves can travel from the nose, mouth or intestine to the central nervous system through the cranial nerves (including the vagus nerve), as well as through other parts of the autonomic nervous system. Microbial products and microbes can also travel through the blood. Note that the pathway is bidirectional. It is also possible for neuronal molecules and microbes to travel from the central nervous system to the nose, mouth, and gut.

It is tempting to suggest that the pathways shown in Figure 5 help us to understand the origin of the various modes of onset of amyotrophic lateral sclerosis (ALS). Some patients develop slurred speech and difficulty swallowing in the early stages of ALS, suggestive of brainstem involvement. This could be because of microbial influences in the nose or mouth. Other people may have onset with weakness in an ankle, which may be because of the influence of microbial factors from the intestine on the spinal cord.

There are more than 100 million neurons in the gastrointestinal tract, more than in the spinal cord. Bacteria and bacterial products can influence these neurons in the gut. Those interactions can be transmitted to the brain through the autonomic nervous system and cause disease. Is there a precedent for this? The answer is yes. It's known that intestinal exposure to proteins with an amyloid configuration can cause a protein-folding disorder in the brain. The best example of this is bovine spongiform encephalopathy (BSE), also known as mad cow disease. This happens when infected beef causes one of the body's proteins to become abnormally folded, leading to rapid neurodegeneration and death. An outbreak of this disorder in the United Kingdom in the 1980s caused over 200 deaths (see Chapter 7). The transmissible agent in this disease is a misfolded protein called a prion. A similar process was discovered in eastern New Guinea in the 1950s, in an epidemic of a brain degeneration called kuru. In this condition, the brain degeneration was caused by an infectious protein transmitted though the eating of a relative's infected brain tissue.[II]

It is believed that the pathway of transmission of the prion from the gut to the brain is through the autonomic nervous system, particularity the vagus nerve. The vagus is a nerve that provides input to the gut from the brain as

[II] Cannibalism in New Guinea declined in the second half of the twentieth century after contact with the Western world was established. The disease is now extinct.

well as input from the brain to the gut. It connects the lower regions of the brain in the brainstem to the intestines and other organs. If we eat too much and feel discomfort, it is because intestinal nerves noted the situation and informed the brain via the vagus. Conversely, if we are hungry and smell dinner and then feel intestinal rumblings, it is because of input from the brain to the gut via the vagus nerve.

The gut–brain pathway involving the vagus nerve has received considerable recent interest.[93] The pathological agent responsible for Parkinson's disease, Alzheimer's disease, or ALS may enter the nervous system through the gut via a prion-like templated misfolding mechanism. Templated refers to the copying of one structure by another, in this case the structure is the folding pattern of a protein. Heiko Braak, a German neuroscientist, and colleagues have demonstrated that the spread of pathology in Parkinson's disease goes from the gut to the brain, as well as from the nose to the brain. The dorsal motor nucleus of the vagus nerve in the medulla is a region affected early in the development of Parkinson's disease and this is where the neurons of origin of the vagus nerve reside. Further evidence for the idea that agents in the gut influence neurodegenerative diseases comes from the observation that people who had their vagus nerve cut in early life, because of peptic ulcer disease, have a lower risk of having Parkinson's disease.[94]

Remarkably, studies show that neurodegenerative disease proteins can progress *in both directions*, from the gut to the brain or from the brain to the gut through the vagus nerve. This describes a bidirectional gut–brain axis (pathway). It has been documented that the gut bacteria modulate brain activity through this axis (see Figure 5). The gut bacteria also produce chemicals such as catecholamines, the neurotransmitter serotonin, and gamma-aminobutyric acid, SCFAs, functional bacterial amyloids, and other agents which affect the functions of the brain.

People often ask me how bacterial products get to the intestinal nervous system, since there is a well-developed and formidable barrier keeping gut contents away from the blood and nerve endings. Although this barrier is an important feature of the gastrointestinal tract, it isn't perfect. There are cells on the lining of the intestine that receive nerve endings containing the Parkinson's disease-related protein alpha-synuclein. There is more alpha-synuclein in the gut than in the brain. The pathway of the gut–brain axis can be involved in brain diseases without requiring the molecules or organisms to travel directly from the gut to the brain. It may be their meta-bolic products which travel through the pathway. It may be that misfolding of neuronal proteins can be initiated in the gut and transmitted to the brain in a manner similar to that of the prion diseases, such as BSE. Furthermore, bacteria and bacterial products in the gut can influence the immune cells which are present there, and these cells are known to travel everywhere in the body, including the brain. Since the microbiota are our most important envi-ronmental exposure, it is necessary for the immune sys-tem to know what is going on in the contents of the gut. It is evolutionarily required that there are mechanisms by which the immune system can sample gut molecules and organisms.

Since the microbiota are our most important environmental exposure, it is necessary for the immune system to know what is going on in the contents of the gut.

Microbiota-Based Treatments for Disease

The potential for the development of preventive and ther-apeutic agents that influence the microbiota is enormous, as these partner organisms are dependent on what we feed them. There are many ways to alter their composition, including diet, prebiotics, probiotics, antibiotics, and fecal microbiota transplant. Prebiotics are foods and other agents that enhance the growth of healthful bacteria. These are usually fiber-containing products, such as indigestible complex carbohydrates (found in root vegetables, greens, fruit, oats, and seeds). Probiotics are live bacteria that have desirable influences on health, such as yogurt or kimchi.

People with an overgrowth of a dangerous bacteria in the gut called *Clostridiodes* (formerly *Clostridium*) *difficile* can die. The disease often doesn't respond to antibiotics. However, many patients have been cured by a process called fecal microbiota transplant (FMT). With FMT, feces are taken from a person who is screened for the absence of infectious diseases and administered to the patient. This procedure significantly changes the bacterial population inside the recipient and has resulted in an excellent cure rate of the infection. Research is under way on expanding the opportunity to repair dysbiosis though bacterial therapies. Proprietary mixtures of bacteria that can be used in place of FMT are being carried out and trials of FMT for Parkinson's disease and ALS are under way. (Live bacterial cocktail therapies may be comprised of as many as 50+ strains.)

These new therapies require close attention to the unique nature of bacterial communities in the body. Since everyone has a different microbiome, therapies will need to be personalized to each person's own microbial ecology. It is estimated that there are twice as many phages (viruses that infect bacteria) in the gut as there are bacteria. Research into the influence of phages on microbial activities in the gut is just beginning. There is potential for specific phages to be engineered to have precise influences on aspects of bacterial communities. It is promising to consider the untapped potential of microbial-based therapies.

As our microbial partners influence so many aspects of our health and fitness, they are intricately involved in protecting us from age-related changes and other threats. They are a critical part of our physical reserve.

9 THE HEALTH OF THE BODY AND THE PHYSICAL RESERVE FACTOR

As we age, we have a little bit less of everything: less energy, less physical flexibility, less learning capacity. That's why the concept of multiple reserve factors is so important.

An example will be helpful. Consider the sad scenario of an 80-year-old woman who falls at home and breaks her hip. She's taken to the hospital for surgery and develops pneumonia and delirium, then dies. (Delirium was discussed in Chapter 5.) This is a common occurrence in hospitals. Her cause of death may be recorded on the death certificate as "bacterial pneumonia," and it may be that she died because she acquired a particularly dangerous strain of bacteria, which was unresponsive to antibiotics. However, there are many other factors that may have contributed to her death. Looking at these multiple possibilities shows the interconnected reserve factors involved in human health.

- Why did she fall? Factors that contribute to falls include alcohol use, depression, social isolation, medications influencing drowsiness, or the presence of unsafe conditions in the home (unstable rugs, electrical cords, pets). Did she fall because of a neurological problem, such as vitamin B12 deficiency (associated with stomach inflammation and vegetarian diet), weakness, or a previous unrecognized stroke?

- Did she have osteoporosis? Perhaps if her bone density had been higher, she would not have had the fracture. Was her bone density low because of medications or because of a calcium-deficient diet? Perhaps she was known to have osteoporosis and had been prescribed calcium supplements but did not take them?
- Did she have a poor immune response to bacteria infecting her lungs? This could be caused by anemia, vitamin C or D deficiency, alcoholism, medications, or malnutrition. When people age, there is impaired production of vitamin D by the skin and vitamin D is important for the functioning of the immune system.
- Did she have an unhealthy population of gut and lung bacteria? The microbiota play an important role in the immune response to disease-causing organisms.
- Did she have a gastrointestinal problem that altered absorption and metabolism of the antibiotics which were prescribed for her pneumonia?
- Was she frail? Frailty is associated with an increased risk of falling, as well as a greater risk of dying from falls or from pneumonia.[95] Older people who are underweight may lack the resources to survive an illness – including falls – where there is little opportunity for nutritional intake. This is because hospitalized patients may not eat well because of cognitive disturbances, depression, poor food quality, isolation, sedating medications, and other factors.
- Did she have a poor diet? Population-based studies have shown that older people at home who eat a less diverse diet than others have a higher risk of frailty.[96]
- Did she have preexisting lung, cardiac, or kidney disease? These diseases increase the chance of getting pneumonia and delirium. When that happens, the chance of dying increases.

- Did she develop delirium because of inappropriate medications (common in older people), preexisting neurodegenerative disease (e.g., early stages of Alzheimer's disease, vascular cognitive impairment), or unrecognized thyroid disease?
- Did a lack of a social support system contribute to a poor diet, which impacted osteoporosis as well as frailty and sensitivity to pneumonia and delirium?
- Did a lack of a social support system contribute to depression and poor medication compliance?
- Was she depressed? Depression is also a risk factor for falls and frailty.
- Did she have a sleep disturbance that led to instability and falling, as well as an increased occurrence of aspiration and pneumonia?
- Did she have medical problems that could not be addressed because of poverty or lack of access to care?
- Was she obese? Obese people suffer impaired immune responses to infections and excessive autoimmunity.
- Did she have a low cognitive reserve, increasing her risk of falling and all of the subsequent consequences of her fall?

More possible interactions could be listed. The complex web of interdependent interactions in this case illustrates the multiple determinants of health and disease. This matter can also be illustrated with a positive outcome. Imagine an 80-year-old woman who does not fall, does not develop pneumonia and delirium, and lives to 96 years of age with meaningful interactions with friends and family. The chance for this desirable outcome will only be enhanced if her bodily and social interactions are working well.

The degree to which there are intact performance abilities in these domains (cognitive, systemic, psychological, and social) is the key to the concept of multiple reserves. The degree to which human performance is affected by declines with age depends upon these interactions.

Aging well isn't just about avoiding death and disease. Aging healthily also means keeping the reserve capacity of our component systems high so that, as function declines with age, performance is less severely affected, and fitness is better maintained. The good news is there are lots of things everyone can do to maximize healthful interactions inside our body and between ourselves and friends, family, and community.

The good news is there are lots of things everyone can do to maximize healthful interactions inside our body and between ourselves and friends, family, and community.

The body's organ systems are interconnected and interdependent. Our muscles are able to contract because of the supply of glucose and oxygen in the blood. Glucose is provided by the gut and the liver, and oxygen by the lungs, with the assistance, of course, of the heart. Our lungs are able to work because of the muscular actions of the chest and diaphragm, blood supplied by the right side of the heart, and the ability of the left side of the heart to accept the blood coming from the lungs. Our immune system maintains our resistance to pathogens and our body's ability to repair damage because of interactions with the microbiota. The immune system also enables the cells in the spleen, liver, and bone marrow to produce the necessary molecules and cellular elements we need. All of these activities are monitored by the brain.

These interdependent activities are critical to aging because of the relatively reduced function of all systems. Imagine a 75 year-old woman who has the early stages of Alzheimer's-related pathology in the brain, with no change in performance. If she also has a reduced cardiac output, low blood sugar, anemia, dehydration, urinary tract infection, polypharmacy (too many or inappropriate medications), poor lung function, alcohol abuse, or other systemic problems, impaired neurological function may develop without any additional damage or injury to the brain.

The brain obviously controls perception, conscious and unconscious emotions, language, and many other nervous system activities. Remarkably, the brain also influences hair growth, heart rhythm, kidney function, digestive enzyme secretion, gastrointestinal tract movements, and myriad other body activities. It is hard to find a human function which is not influenced by the brain. The brain is also dependent on the other body parts. It requires nearly constant supply of blood, oxygen, and glucose. Because of these continuous needs it is reliant upon the bone marrow producing red blood cells, the heart pumping blood, the arteries delivering the correct amount of blood, the liver producing a constant supply of glucose at correct levels, and the kidneys regulating electrolyte concentrations and water balance.

It needs to be a goal of our aging to enhance the possibility that negative interactions do not take place.

It needs to be a goal of our aging to enhance the possibility that negative interactions do not take place. In order to pursue this goal, we need to manage our lifestyle activities so that our fitness levels can be enhanced. By this I mean fitness in the sense of interdependence – fitness of all the body parts, not only one of them.

The Role of Our Organ Systems in Brain Health and Fitness with Aging

Let's review what are some of the ways in which systemic factors influence the brain.

Defense against Infectious Disease

Two people of the same age may acquire disease-causing microbes in the same part of the body with the same organism and with the same dose of pathogens and have vastly different results. The ability to resist the infection depends upon the ability of the multiple reserves to maintain a state of healthy balance (homeostasis). The potential for disease caused by an infectious agent is related to nutritional status, body weight, immune competency, and the microbiota. An inadequate immune response, related to vitamin and other nutritional deficiencies, may lead to disability or death.

On the other hand, an excessive response to an infection may have deleterious effects on the body. This situation, which is more common in older than younger persons, develops when the immune response to pathogens causes damage exceeding the damage caused by the infectious agent. This has been observed in viral and bacterial meningitis and encephalitis, as well as viral pneumonia, including coronavirus disease 2019 (Covid-19).[97] The propensity to develop these excessive responses is influenced by the composition of the microbiome. The process of excessive immune responses may involve a lack of tolerance. We are home to several trillion of our microbial partners, and it is critical that the immune system's surveillance does not lead to an attack on organisms that we need to tolerate (not attack). Our capacity for tolerance is set by the microbiota.

Infectious disorders anywhere in the body can negatively influence brain function. Inflammation anywhere in the body has been associated with cognitive impairment as well as strokes, small brain hemorrhages, Alzheimer's disease, Parkinson's disease, and amyotrophic lateral sclerosis (ALS).[98]

The Microbiota and the Gastrointestinal Tract

The role of the microbiota is critical in these interactions amongst our organ systems. As discussed in the previous chapter, gut bacteria that like to eat meat, cheese, and eggs (meat cheese and eggs contain carnitine, choline, and phosphatidylcholine) enhance the growth of bacteria that make a molecule called trimethylamine (TMA). (There is more carnitine in red meat then in chicken or fish.) TMA is oxidized in the liver to trimethylamine oxide (TMAO). This molecule has been found in elegant studies from the Cleveland Clinic to accelerate impairment of cardiac and brain blood vessels, leading to heart attacks and stroke. TMAO increases the propensity of platelets to stick to the blood vessel wall and increases the deposition of lipids in the blood vessels. Serum TMAO has also been found to be increased in Alzheimer's disease and mild cognitive impairment.[75] People on vegetarian diets have bacteria that produce less TMAO. This work is being explored for the development of agents to alter the production of TMA by the microbiota. Also, these molecules may be produced in the mouth as well as in the intestine and could have a direct influence on the brain through the cranial nerves and blood vessels.

Our microbiota also protect us from harmful bacteria by occupying unique environmental locations referred to as niches. Their presence in their niche, which may be in the mouth, nose, larynx, pharynx, outer ear, intestinal tract, on the skin, and elsewhere, makes it difficult for disease-causing bacteria to gain a foothold. The "good" bacteria also produce molecules that impair the growth of other bacteria, and they increase the security of the intestinal barrier, which keeps intestinal contents out of the blood.

In order to avoid dysbiosis (an unhealthy state of the gut bacteria) we need to have a high-fiber, diverse diet. Beware of the risk factors that diminish the multiple reserve factors (see Chapter 5).

Endocrine System
Adult-onset diabetes is a significant risk factor for Alzheimer's disease and cognitive impairment caused by stroke.

If you have diabetes, don't fret. There are things you can do to live a healthier life: diet and exercise are key. So is managing obesity. A high-fiber diet may improve insulin responsiveness, which helps in the management of diabetes. The influence of diabetes on cognition is complex, as the condition contributes to vascular damage in the brain, which also increases dementia risk. Both the high- and low-blood-sugar episodes in diabetes may contribute to loss of cognition. People with diabetes also have an impaired resistance to infection together with a risk of peripheral neuropathy, peripheral vascular disease, and kidney impairment. There are persons with diabetes who may remove their diabetic state by loss of weight, exercise, and dietary changes.

Thyroid deficiency is also common in older persons and can cause cognitive losses.

Body Weight and Metabolism

Obesity is a risk factor for cognitive impairment, stroke, and Alzheimer's disease. There are negative effects of obesity on the structure and function of the cortex of the brain in aging. These matters may be related to complex interactions of obesity with other factors, such as diabetes, hypertension, poor diet, and less physical activity. Obese persons have an overactive immune system, which can have damaging effects on age-related brain conditions. Regarding the association of obesity with immune hyperactivation, obesity is like having an active wound. Body weight is not the only matter of concern. Abdominal deposition of adipose tissue (fat) is associated with several poor health outcomes.

It is also unhealthy to be significantly underweight. For persons aged 65 years and older it may be more hazardous to their health to be underweight than overweight. People who are underweight lack nutritional reserves that can sustain them during an illness or other stressful episode.

The development of frailty is also a danger for under-weight persons. A recent study in the Democratic Republic of the Congo showed that young adults who had experienced severe acute malnutrition in childhood were at risk for deficits in educational attainment and cognitive function when they grew older.[99]

Hypertension

Hypertension (high blood pressure) in middle age is an important risk factor for the development of Alzheimer's disease in later life. It is a key risk factor for cardiovascular and cerebral vascular disease as well. Hypertension may lead to small or large strokes, as well as vascular damage to the white matter, which can cause significant cognitive impairment. Control of hypertension is vital for people of all ages.

Sensory Deficits

It's easy to overlook the eyes and ears, but don't do it. Visual and auditory problems are both common with aging and can hasten the appearance of cognitive impairment, Alzheimer's disease, and depression. Hearing problems disturb communication and may lead to loneliness and depression. Hearing loss is one of the most modifiable risk factors for dementia and may be responsible for 9 percent of cases.[100] Research supports the value of cataract repair and the use of hearing aids in improving behavioral performance. Certainly, it is important that the risk of sensory deficits is reduced, through the recognition and management of glaucoma and the avoidance of sound-induced trauma to the ears. Sensory deficits can play an important role in restricting social and physical activities, with negative consequences for the brain.

If you love listening to the Beatles or George Frideric Handel with the volume cranked to eleven, don't. Exposure to loud noises for long periods of time elicit harmful stress responses linked to depression and cognitive impairment, as well as heart disease. Furthermore, noise-induced trauma to the inner ear can cause the permanent loss of hearing ability.

Frailty

Frailty is a condition of increased vulnerability caused by decreased physical capacity. When this happens, there is an impaired response to stress.[100] Frailty is a common condition in older persons, with an increased risk for poor health outcomes such as falls, dementia, delirium, depression, hospitalization, and mortality. Frailty can have both physical and psychological effects. It is also linked to cognitive impairment and delirium and is associated with more rapid decline and a higher conversion rate from mild cognitive impairment to Alzheimer's disease.

Heart and Lungs

Good heart and lung health is linked closely to good brain health. This is clearly because both the heart and the brain share blood vessel systems with similar characteristics. One academic paper emphasized this with the title, "Healthy young hearts sharper older minds make."[101]

As mentioned above, hypertension in midlife is a risk factor for cognitive impairment in later life, through the increased risk of both Alzheimer's disease and stroke. Failing pump function of the heart lowers blood pressure and brain perfusion and can cause cognitive impairment, and atrophy of the brain. Atrial fibrillation as well as valvular heart disease can cause strokes. Chronic obstructive pulmonary disease (also called emphysema) can impair cerebral circulation and cause cognitive impairment and strokes.

Anemia (a low amount of red blood cells in the circulation) is associated with an increased risk of Alzheimer's disease, cognitive impairment without Alzheimer's disease, white matter degeneration, and cerebral microbleeds. One study found that the risk of developing dementia was increased by 34 percent by the presence of anemia. Older persons with the highest and lowest hemoglobin levels have a higher risk of dementia and cognitive decline.

Kidneys

There is good evidence for an association between kidney dysfunction and cognitive impairment and dementia. Evidence suggests that albumin in the urine is associated with higher odds of developing cognitive impairment or dementia and reduced kidney function predicts disability.[24] Chronic kidney disease has been linked to white matter disease and cognitive impairment.

Liver

The liver plays an essential role in the body's regulatory activities. It removes toxins and aids the digestion and absorption of nutrients as well as managing glucose supplies, the storage of glycogen, the destruction of red blood cells, and the production of hormones. If the liver is not working properly, toxic products (some made by the microbiota in the gastrointestinal tract) may accumulate in the circulation and damage brain function. The liver produces proteins that bind drugs and other molecules to allow for proper distribution and clearance. One such protein, albumin, helps maintain the balance of fluids in our tissues and circulation, and also transports molecules in the blood, such as hormones, enzymes, and vitamins. In a 2010 study, we found that low albumin levels are associated with a higher risk of cognitive impairment.[102]

Protection from Environmental and Self-Made (Endogenous) Toxins

The liver, kidneys, and the microbiota all play crucial roles in detoxifying environmental toxins as well as those made by the body. It is important that they be in good shape throughout life because they are so important for our physical reserve.

Oral Health

Periodontitis is a risk factor for heart disease and stroke as well as Alzheimer's disease. Studies show that oral bacteria produce proteins that increase the risk of large and small bleeding in the brain.[73] Also, loss of teeth is associated with cognitive impairment and Alzheimer's disease. There is a lack of convincing evidence that mercury in amalgam dental fillings is a risk factor for Alzheimer's disease.

Response to Surgery

Older persons and those with cognitive impairment and Alzheimer's disease are more sensitive to the negative effects of anesthetic agents and of surgical procedures. The risk for postoperative delirium is higher in cognitively impaired subjects. Everyone should be aware of the risks of surgery and it should only be done when absolutely necessary.

Pain

Chronic pain can cause cognitive impairment in many ways: depression, social isolation, impaired physical activity, toxicity of medications, and systemic inflammation. In addition, the effects of chronic stress can damage the brain.

Comorbidities

Many older people suffer from multiple conditions at the same time. The impact of medical illnesses on brain function is more than additive. Having more than one chronic condition is bad. And worse than you think. Multiple chronic conditions often have more impact on function that expected from each condition alone.

A 2014 study showed that, among Medicare beneficiaries with dementia, 38 percent had comorbid coronary artery disease, 37 percent had diabetes, 29 percent had chronic kidney disease, 28 percent had congestive heart failure, and 25 percent had chronic obstructive pulmonary disease.[103]

Conclusion

A friend of mine recently suffered a tragedy in his family. His 74-year-old father was in good health and suffered knee pain from chronic arthritis. He was advised to have knee replacement surgery and elected to have both knees replaced at the same time, despite pleas from his family to do them one at a time. He wished to have the associated disability and pain over with as soon as possible and would not change his mind about having the knees replaced on one day. Three days after surgery he developed pneumonia and subsequently died. Major surgery is a severe stress to the balance of bodily functions. At the age of 74, his physical reserve factor was less than it had been when he was younger.

Had I been consulted, I would have objected to the idea of having both knees replaced at one time. It is valuable to remember that the physical reserve factor is lower in older persons. Often, we don't have a choice about what forms of stress we are exposed to. When we do have a choice, we should be careful to respect our limitations. Also, through our lifestyle activities we should strive to enhance our physical reserve factor so that we can have the best possible response to both predicted and unpredicted stresses.

10 DEPRESSION, ANXIETY, AND WHAT GOOD IS FEELING BAD?

> *Why are so many of us constantly anxious, spending our lives, as Mark Twain said, "suffering from tragedies that never occur"?*
>
> Randolph Nesse, American physician, and cofounder of the field of evolutionary medicine

Viktor Frankl, Austrian psychoanalyst, and author of the exceptionally important book *Man's Search for Meaning*, once had a patient who was stressed out about work. A diplomat, the patient struggled with a demanding boss. The diplomat's previous analyst had tried to convince him that his unhappiness was tied to an underlying resentment of his father. After the death of the analyst, the patient came to see Frankl. After a few visits, Frankl determined that the patient's difficulties were because his job "frustrated his will to meaning." Frankl advised the patient to leave the job, which he did. After he quit his job, his main psychological problems were quickly resolved. Of course, the story simplifies a complex process, but it does illustrate the reality that emotional states may result from life situations in need of repair.

Depression may be a warning sign of mental or physical illness, or, as in the case of Frankl's patient, a sign of a troubled working environment. Recognizing the presence of depression is key to dealing with it effectively.

Awareness of Depression

Depression is common in older people. People who are depressed may have significant memory problems. The recurrent thought of sadness and regret seen in depression may interfere with the registration of new memories. It can develop as a response to life events and appear independently of what is happening. People with a history of serious and recurrent depression may experience more depression with age. However, people who didn't experience depression in their younger years may also develop depression without any history of previous sad emotions.

Is everyone with depression aware of its presence? How can persons and family members be aware of its appearance? Many depressed older persons are aware of their depression, but some are not. It is common that a spouse or other loved one may be aware of a person's depression while the person denies it. Depression may also be present without the awareness of anyone in the family. This may be because someone has grown up in an environment in which feelings were not respected. This situation is especially common for persons who were young in times of poverty because their parents were overwhelmed trying to cope with the situation. It's important to seek help at all ages because effective treatments are available.

Signs of depression include, of course, sadness and recurring thoughts of regret. Depression is also indicated by loss of appetite, loss of weight, difficulty with sleeping, loss of interest in activities, and loss of interest in sexual activities. These so-called vegetative signs of depression may also be caused by other conditions: loss of appetite and loss of weight can be signs of cancer, deficient thyroid hormones, or other systemic illness. The presence of these signs may be of value nonetheless to suggest the consideration of depression.

Depression and Other Illnesses

Depression may be associated with cerebral vascular disease, such as small and large strokes and the loss of integrity of the white matter of the brain. Changes in the microbiota have also been observed in persons with depression, and interventions aimed at changing the gut bacteria may help. Transplantation of the gut bacteria from humans with depression to animals has been found to induce depression-like behaviors. It is also crucial to appreciate the physical factors that can create or enhance depression, including poor sleep, deficiency of vitamins B12, B6 (pyridoxine), low thyroid function, and deficiency of folic acid.

Depression is a risk factor for dementia as well as heart disease and can be caused and worsened by sleep disorders, as well as systemic illness.

Depression is a risk factor for dementia as well as heart disease and can be caused and worsened by sleep disorders, as well as systemic illness. People with depression and anxiety also have an earlier onset of Alzheimer's disease compared to those without such a history.

Depression and What We Do

The ability to manage our response to life events is a fundamental part of our psychological reserve factor. Depression can be caused or aggravated by a lack of social interactions and physical activity. It may be linked to life events and may also be completely independent of them.

Several lifestyle behaviors may be associated with the development of depression. Many persons have replaced social interaction with television and social media. Excessive television viewing can enhance depression because it does not allow for participation and floods the brain with more stimuli than can possibly be processed. This is done while the television is telling viewers there is a crisis and they must pay attention. One US cable news network features a program called "Breaking News." Such a title implies that there is something of extraordinary importance. This certainly does happen, as it did on September 11, 2001. But for most of the time we do not need to be overly attentive to world events, and we should not be monstrously worried all the time about everything. Also, a television advertisment may show a millisecond clip of a person being stabbed, followed by an explosion, followed by someone falling from an airplane. The brain is only capable of handling a certain amount of visual information each second. Often, the stimuli are delivered at a rate that can't possibly be processed by the human brain. And there is no opportunity for interaction. This supersaturation of our sensory processes can lead to negative emotional states. This is a special problem for older people who may have fewer opportunities to seek activities other than television.

Social media can also induce negative emotional states. The content of Facebook and Instagram posts is often a constant and painful reminder of the happy lives of other people. An important message from other people's curated photos of themselves at family events, restaurants, and outdoor activities is that they are living a happy, perfect life. This just isn't so. Very few people post photos of themselves lying around on the sofa doing nothing, visiting the dentist, or having a colonoscopy. Randolph Nesse, cited above, said:[104] "The kinds of attention we get on social media is really very much like crack cocaine. We have social obesity I call it – we can't stop our consumption of opportunities to display ourselves and get feedback from other people." If social media sites like Facebook, Instagram, TikTok, and Snapchat irritate you, stop using them.

The relationship of depression to our activities has the nature of a "vicious cycle." Inactivity leads to depression, fatigue, and apathy. And depression leads to inactivity and lack of energy. It is more accurate to consider these interactions as a "vicious spiral," as the effects are cumulative and get worse with time. Let's consider how to turn these processes into a "virtuous cycle," a repeating cycle of events, each increasing the beneficial effect of the other. If activity increases, depression may be relieved, leading to more activity that helps to resolve depression.

It can help if we first address the basic question of why we are capable of depression. Depression can also result from infection in the body anywhere, with the production of immune molecules that may enter the brain.[105] If you have an illness like influenza and are confined to bed for several days, you may have noted the onset of depression caused, in part, by inactivity.

It is harder to be depressed when you're active. Our ancestors, who lived in very different environments to the ones we have today, needed to rest when sick or injured. Through natural selection, a program of behaviors has developed to enhance the chance that we will rest if our health is challenged (called sickness behavior). About 10,000 years ago, an ancestor of ours with an infection would be wise to not go hunting, but rather to rest. This evolutionary consideration is responsible, in part, for the feelings of depression, headache, and malaise that accompany fever in infectious illnesses. Interferon is a molecule produced in the body in response to viral disorders. Headache is one of its common side effects, perhaps because it may be an evolutionary guide to help us to rest.

So depression may be an adaptive response to systemic illness, as it encourages inactivity, which may be a helpful response to the illness.

Mental Health and Aging

Depression can have a big influence on our multiple reserve factors. There is evidence that exposure to physical and emotional stress in early life, including post-traumatic stress disorder (PTSD), is a risk factor for cognitive impairment, hypertension, and depression in later life. In a Swedish study of more than 61,000 people, those who had experienced PTSD showed a 31 percent increased risk of neurodegenerative disease and an 81 percent increased risk of vascular cognitive impairment.[106]

Mental health is especially important as we age. Henry Krystal, psychiatrist and Holocaust survivor, noted how the psychological work, conscious and unconscious, needed to deal with traumatic experiences can become fragmented in later life.[28,107] "Old age, with its losses," Krystal said, "imposes the inescapable necessity to face one's past. This development determines that one either accepts oneself and one's past or continues to reject it angrily."

In other words, the choice is, as the child psychiatrist Erik Erikson put it, of "integration or despair."[29] With aging, there is often a shift from thinking and planning to remembering, a change which can be difficult if the early life events were traumatic. People may have spent a lifetime fighting against recalling painful experiences in early life, and this process may become difficult with age.

Aspects of the psychological and social reserve factors related to depression include isolation, loneliness, poverty, inactivity, apathy, malnutrition, sensory deficits, and poor access to healthcare. It has been observed in transgenic Alzheimer model mice that social isolation exacerbates memory deficits and increases deposits of the amyloid-beta protein in the brain. One study found the risk of Alzheimer's disease to be double in persons with loneliness compared to those without. Feeling lonely may be accompanied by thoughts of emptiness or rejection and is a sign of social isolation.

The presence of larger social networks is protective of cognitive function in older people and enhances all the reserves. However, such networks are often impaired by aging. The beneficial effects of social interactions are not limited to the brain. They provide mental stimulation, which enhances cognitive reserve, as well as physical activity, which improves physical reserve. Active participation in the life of the world is good for us at all stages of life.

Why Are We Capable of Sad Thoughts?

Depressed persons have impaired performance. Why has evolution permitted the generation of this negative emotional state? The answer is suggested by the essay entitled, "What good is feeling bad?" by physician Randolph Nesse, a founder of the field of evolutionary medicine.[104] He asserts that depression is not a citalopram-deficiency disease. That is, depression is not caused by a lack of antidepressant medication. Depression may have many causes and some of them can be remediated without drugs. We have evolved the capacity for experiencing depression because it may have adaptive value. Depression can be a sign that there is something wrong which needs to be remedied (as suggested by the story of Victor Frankl's patient at the beginning of the chapter).

We have evolved the capacity for experiencing depression because it may have adaptive value.

The ability of health professionals to learn about patients' lives is a critical issue because physicians tend to be busy and may not always have the time, or interest, to learn about what may be causing a patient's depression. It takes 60 seconds to prescribe an antidepressant and 60 minutes or more to learn about the emotional life of a person.

According to Nesse, "Rather than assuming that negative feelings are symptoms of a physical abnormality or a dysfunctional personality, family or society, the therapist can consider the possibility that some suffering is part of a vital mechanism shaped by natural selection to help people survive in the environment."[104] Our capacity to feel depression and anxiety has evolved because these feelings may help us endure, in a similar manner to the value of physical pain, which enhances our defenses against injury. Just as we use physical pain as a guide to behavior, we may need to use depression as a sign that corrective actions are needed.

What Can We Do about Depression?

Depression can be well treated with a wide variety of medications which can be highly effective, although older persons shouldn't take antidepressants that impair cholinergic neurotransmission, such as nortriptyline or imipramine. A wide range of major tranquilizers should also be avoided such as trifluoperazine, chlorpromazine, and others (see Chapter 23). There are modern antidepressants available which have fewer side effects and good efficacy. Counseling with psychiatrists, psychologists, or social workers may be very helpful.

While rest is important during illness, our lives should be filled with vigorous physical activity. The natural state of humans is to be physically active. A lack of physical activity can precipitate and worsen depression. Physical exercise improves one's emotional state. We are not by nature made to be sedentary creatures.

Physical exercise in some form or other is within the capacity of most people and should be pursued as if life depended on it, because it does. Running, walking, swimming, and other physical activities not only help avoid depression, but also delay age-related cognitive impairment and improve performance in people with mild cognitive impairment.[108] A lack of exercise is a known risk factor for early death as well as coronary heart disease, stroke, and diabetes.

I hope that the realization that aging is not inevitable is helpful in appreciating with gratitude the opportunity presented by aging. As remarked by William James (yes, him again), "The greatest weapon against stress is our ability to choose one thought over another."

"The greatest weapon against stress is our ability to choose one thought over another."

A favorite thought experiment of mine is to consider what the dead would say if they had the chance. How would they respond if told that we are upset because of the rain or because our favorite team lost a game? I imagine that they would have a stern admonishment for us and tell us to appreciate the immense value of life.

11 GENETICS AREN'T EVERYTHING

Genetics loads the gun ... environment pulls the trigger.
Dr. Francis Collins, Genetics researcher and Former Director
of the US National Institutes of Health

A married couple, both university professors in their 50s, were concerned about their prospects of developing Alzheimer's disease as they aged. They didn't have a notable family history of dementing illness and had no signs of cognitive illness. Without any professional guidance, they were tested for the presence or absence of the most important Alzheimer's risk gene, apolipoprotein E (APOE). Their genes were tested and both were found to have one apolipoprotein E ε4 gene (allele). Their 28-year-old daughter was also intellectually curious and was tested and was found, unfortunately, to have two APOE ε4 alleles, meaning that her risk of developing Alzheimer's later in life is more than 10 times higher, compared to people without any ε4 alleles. Currently there is nothing she can do with this information (except worry). There is no specific intervention designed to diminish the influence of the APOE ε4 allele on development of Alzheimer's disease. Furthermore, it is estimated that about 40–50 percent of people who have two copies of the APOE ε4 allele at the age of 80 do not have dementia. It is conceivable that she will worry about her high risk of developing Alzheimer's disease for the next 52 years and then learn at the age of 80 that she hasn't gotten it after all. How will she explain this to current or future partners?

I am concerned that many people will have themselves tested for the APOE ε4 gene because of new opportunities to obtain genetic testing, but won't make use of genetic counseling. The data concerning risk of this and other genes are complex, and undoubtedly many persons (as well as many physicians) do not appreciate this complexity. When a medical intervention is developed based on knowing the APOE genotype, it will be clearly important for people to be tested. However, this is not the case at the moment. Persons considering having this testing done should discuss the situation with an informed physician and determine if the information obtained will enhance or diminish their quality of life.

There are things that can be done to lower the risk of developing dementia (reviewed in Chapters 5 and 12). These are things everyone can and should do. Everyone has a risk of getting dementing illness with age. Many people get Alzheimer's disease even though they do not possess an APOE ε4 gene. In short, genetic tests aren't needed to increase commitment to preventive measures.

What Is Our Genetic Makeup and How Does It Influence Our Lives?

Humans are born with 23 pairs of chromosomes and 20,000–25,000 genes. Genes are sequences of nucleotides (the basic structural unit of nucleic acids) that code for the amino acid sequence of proteins. With the exception of our gonads (testicles and ovaries), all of our cells have the same DNA. It is important to know that the genetic information contained in the chromosomes does not directly determine what happens to us. Rather, the genes provide information about what can be done. What actually happens is an interaction between the genes and the environment. That is, how we live influences the action of our genes.

How we live influences the action of our genes.

To put it another way, the context is supreme: Dr. Mina Bissel, Iranian American breast cancer researcher, said:[109] "The sequence of the genes are [sic] like the keys on the piano. It is the context that makes the music." The cells in my hair follicles that make hair have the same genes as the cells in my pancreas that make insulin. The activity of the cell is determined by both the genes and the environmental stimuli.

A good example of this is what happens when a bone is fractured, and a cast applied. After several weeks of enforced rest, the muscles on the arm, which have not been active, will become smaller (this process is called atrophy). When the cast is removed, and the muscles are able to work again, they will grow back to normal size. Without activity, muscle cells make few new proteins and atrophy develops (the genes for making protein are not being used, the genes are not being expressed). When the muscle is used again, genes for making the protein become active. In this case it is the environmental demand which determines which genes are active in the cell (or which notes are played on the piano).

The relationship of the work of genes to environmental demands is also illustrated by the detoxication of alcohol. Some people will begin to feel drowsy with just half a glass of wine. Others can consume one-half of a bottle or more and retain wakefulness. The difference, at least in part, is the production of proteins called microsomal oxidizing enzymes, which are made by the liver and detoxify alcohol, lowering the alcohol level in the blood. The more one drinks alcohol, the more that the genes for this enzyme are activated, and more of the enzyme is produced. If a person who has a limited capacity for staying awake after a small dose of alcohol was to gradually increase their intake, they could develop a greater level of expression of these enzymes, so that higher levels of alcohol could be drunk without drowsiness. (This is mentioned purely as a demonstration of the concept of gene expression being related to the environment. Don't try this at home!)

Another example of the importance of gene–environment interactions is phenylketonuria (PKU), which was one of the commonest causes of inherited mental disability. It is caused by a genetic defect in the ability to metabolize phenylalanine, an amino acid found in food. Subjects with PKU develop high levels of phenylalanine in the blood, which is toxic to the brain.

However, when the PKU diagnosis is established at birth, the diet can be adjusted so that toxic levels of the amino acid never appear, and the person has no neurological damage. The gene cannot at present be repaired, but the result of the genetic defect can be bypassed through an environmental change. Similarly, some people have a family history of early cardiac death, which may be due to genetic abnormalities that lead to high levels of lipids in the blood (hyperlipidemia). With the management of lifestyle factors, including the control of hypertension, not smoking, avoidance of obesity, exercise, a low-fat diet, and lipid-lowering statin drugs, these persons may have a long and healthy lifespan, even though their defective genetic code can't be repaired (at least at the moment).

Humans have become significantly taller in the twenty-first century than in prior centuries. There are strong genetic influences on height, but it is not possible that the genes for height have changed in the past 100 to 200 years. We are taller today because of enhanced nutrition in childhood. As a result, more people are able to reach their genetic height. It has been found that height is inversely correlated to the risk of dementia in Japan (short people are relatively more likely to develop dementia in later life than taller persons). This is most likely because short people are more likely to have been nutritionally deprived in early life, which may have caused them to not reach their genetic height, and also develop less cognitive reserve because of nutritional deficiency.

Genes and Alzheimer's Disease

There are well over 100 different genetic mutations that cause early-onset Alzheimer's disease. These mutations are found on chromosome 1, 14, and 21 and usually cause dementia beginning before the age of 60 and sometimes as early as in the 40s. These mutations are autosomal dominant, meaning that men and women are affected equally and only one copy of the affected gene is required. The mutations are highly penetrant, as people who have the mutation are very likely to get the disease if they live long enough. The molecular information revealed by these mutations has been used to develop therapies to prevent and treat these diseases. However, these experimental treatments have not yet demonstrated success in disease modification. About 99 percent of persons with Alzheimer's disease do not have a mutation in any of these genes.

As noted at the beginning of this chapter, there is another gene that is highly related to the risk of developing Alzheimer's disease. APOE, which is found on chromosome 19, is codominant, which means it is expressed on both the maternal and paternal 19th chromosomes. There are three main forms (alleles) of this gene, referred to as ε2, ε3, or ε4.[110] Therefore, six combinations are possible (ε2/ε2, ε2/ε3, ε2/ε4, ε3/ε3, ε3/ε4, and ε4/ε4). People possessing one copy of the ε4 genotype of APOE have a risk of developing Alzheimer's disease, which is increased about three times than for people having no ε4 allele (see Figure 6).

People who have two copies of the ε4 allele, which is uncommon, have about a 12-fold increased risk of developing the disease, compared to people without an APOE ε4 allele. People with the ε4 allele may also have an earlier onset of the disease than those without the allele. The period of increased risk associated with the APOE ε4 allele begins when they are in their 50s and the increase in risk is higher in women than in men. The additional risk of Alzheimer's disease for those with the ε4 allele decreases after the age of 80. People with two copies of the ε4 allele (homozygotes) have a lifetime risk for Alzheimer's disease of more than 50 percent and for people with one copy of the ε4 allele the lifetime risk is 20–30 percent. People without any copy of ε4 have a lifetime risk of 11 percent for men and 14 percent for women.[111]

But don't despair. In one study, 13 out of 19 people aged 85 years with the ε4/ε4 genotype did not have dementia.

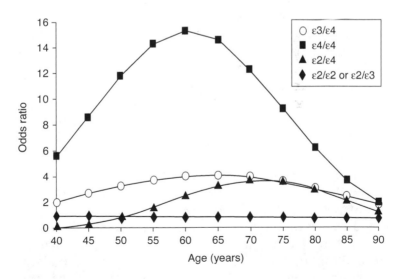

Figure 6 Relative odds of Alzheimer's disease according to APOE genotype and age in Caucasian subjects. The odds ratios are relative to the ε3/ε3 genotype. (Adapted from reference 110.)

This is because the ε4 gene does not cause the disease, it increases the risk. Also, it is common that people with Alzheimer's disease do not possess an ε4 allele (they do not have the risk factor gene).

Why does the APOE gene increase the risk of Alzheimer's disease? We don't know. Several theories have proposed a role for the APOE protein in binding the amyloid-beta protein and enhancing its removal from the brain. The APOE protein is also involved in the security of the blood–brain barrier. As the main role of the protein in the body is to bind lipids, it is likely that this gene's effects on lipid metabolism are involved in the increased risk of Alzheimer's disease.

The APOE gene also has important influences on inflammation. I have been studying the idea that the APOE genotype influences the risk of Alzheimer's disease because of effects of the gene on the gut microbiota. We know that the APOE protein influences lipid binding, and thus may affect the production of mucus in the gut as well as bile acids by the liver. In 2015, I proposed that the gene's influence on the Alzheimer's risk may be because the ε4 form of the gene promotes the growth of unhealthful bacteria in the gut.[57] Recent evidence from a European study supports this hypothesis.[112] This is important because it suggests ways the microbiota can be altered to reduce the risk of Alzheimer's disease.

One unanswered question about the risk from APOE is why it has survived natural selection. Since the ε4 form of the gene is associated with bad outcomes (Alzheimer's disease, stroke, poor recovery from head injury) you might expect that it would have been eliminated by evolution over millennia. In a 2013 paper, my colleagues and I showed that the ε4 form impairs the ability of the malaria parasite to replicate in the blood. This suggests that the ε4 allele may have survived the negative pressure of being associated with disease in late life because it is has a more potent protective effect on survival in early life.

To review, the autosomal-dominant genes that cause Alzheimer's disease are highly penetrant (nearly everyone with the genes develop disease). APOE, on the other hand, is not a causative gene but rather one that increases the risk. It is hoped that one day we will understand why the APOE ε4 allele is associated with Alzheimer's disease, and that a specific therapy can be designed to prevent, delay, or modify the disease. When that happens, it will be clearly indicated for people to be tested to determine their APOE genotype. But, at the moment, information about APOE genotype does not assist us in guiding therapy.

Genes Do Not Work in Isolation

In the scientific community, we are often told that everything is in the genes. In 1975, David Baltimore was awarded the Nobel Prize in Physiology or Medicine for research relating to tumor viruses. In the Siddhartha Mukherjee film on his book, *the Gene*, Baltimore says, "What we've discovered is that everything in biology is genes. We think with genes. We have disease with genes, and so fighting disease by fighting genes makes sense."

This narrow view is wrong. Genes don't work alone, but are able to influence function through their interactions with the environment. It is desirable, of course, to be able to correct abnormal genes through biotechnology. We must not forget another avenue for therapy: we can alter gene–environment interactions to preserve health and fitness.

We must not forget another avenue for therapy: we can alter gene–environment interactions to preserve health and fitness.

It's estimated that genetic factors are involved in 60–80 percent of the risk of getting Alzheimer's disease. As we have noted, people possessing two copies of the APOE ε4 genotype have a much higher risk of getting the disease than people without that form of the gene. However, many people have the disease-associated variant and don't get the disease, and many people who develop Alzheimer's disease do not have the APOE ε4 allele. The role of environmental factors in Alzheimer's is supported by a new study of 96 pairs of monozygotic ("identical") twins who were 60 years of age or older and not cognitively impaired. The study found 14 twin pairs where one twin had molecular signs of Alzheimer's processes in the brain while the other didn't, suggesting that environmental factors are important.[113] This finding underscores the importance of environmental factors, particularly our most important environmental exposure, the microbiota.

There are several genes other than APOE which contribute to Alzheimer's risk. The cumulative effect of these genes is relatively small, compared to the influence of APOE. Another Alzheimer's-related gene is TREM2 (triggering receptor expressed on myeloid cells 2), which normally has an anti-inflammatory influence on the brain. There are rare variants of this gene that have a decreased function, which enhances the risk of Alzheimer's disease. The relationship of this gene to the disease is further evidence in support of the role of the immune system in the disease.

There are also autosomal-dominant genes that cause Parkinson's disease, which are responsible for about 10 percent of cases. Autosomal-dominant genes are also responsible for many cases of frontal temporal lobar degeneration (FTLD), especially when the onset age is below 65 years. One form of FTLD can be caused by a mutation in chromosome

9, called C9ORF72, which can also cause amyotrophic lateral sclerosis (ALS). This mutation can cause either FTLD or ALS, or both in the same person (see Case Study 8). It is not known why some people with this mutation develop ALS, others develop FTLD, and others develop both disorders. Knowledge of these mutations has aided the development of experimental therapies for these conditions, as well as others. The mutations may impair the immune system's ability to interact with the microbiota.

Case Study 8

A 51-year-old patient of mine had cognitive decline for one year, with wandering, falls, and restriction of motion in both hands. He had trouble finding words, was laughing inappropriately, could not do simple calculations, and had reduced strength with loss of muscle mass. He needed help with bathing and could not take care of himself. When asked why he was in the hospital he said that his "computer didn't work." His father died of a brain tumor at the age of 42 and his father's sister had early-onset dementia at the age of 50 with ALS and died when she was 62. Her son also had early-onset dementia with ALS and died at 51. The paternal grandfather also had dementia.

An MRI scan of the brain showed diffuse atrophy (shrinkage) of the cortex, especially in the frontal lobes. A positron emission tomography (PET) scan showed anterior frontal and temporal loss of metabolism. Genetic testing showed a mutation in a gene on chromosome 9, called C9ORF72, which is caused by an abnormal number of repeats in a sequence of guanine (G) and cytosine (C) nucleotides [GGGGCC]. This sequence of six nucleotides is normally repeated only a handful of times, but in this mutation the sequence may be repeated hundreds of times. This mutation was discovered in 2011 and is associated with autosomal-dominant inheritance and the early onset of either FTLD or ALS, or both.

This man clearly had both disorders. This case illustrates a disease that is surely caused by a mutation in a gene. Doctors have observed that the C9ORF72 gene is involved in the functioning of the immune system. Perhaps the mutated gene alters the relationship between the immune system and the microbiota to cause neurodegeneration. It is not known why the same gene can cause two different diseases in members of the same family. It is also not known why the extra number of copies of this particular sequence of six nucleotides is so hazardous.

Scientific inquires continue to investigate the molecular mechanisms involved in this genetic disorder so that treatments can be developed. Genetic cases are responsible for about 10 percent of all cases of ALS and FTLD.

Conclusions

The fact that many people who have one or two copies of ε4 do not get Alzheimer's shows that there must be further interactions responsible for occurrence of disease. This interaction could be between the APOE gene and another gene, or between the APOE gene and environmental factors. And of course it can also be an interaction of several genes and several environmental factors. It is a mistake to believe that the development of Alzheimer's disease in a person with one or two copies of ε4 is caused by the APOE alteration alone.

As we have seen, there are important genetic factors that are responsible for causing Alzheimer's disease. Autosomal-dominant mutations are responsible for only about 1 percent of persons with the disease. For the other 99 percent of cases there isn't an early-onset causative mutation and the disease is not caused by a gene. It is in this majority of cases where it may be possible to avoid "pulling the trigger" and prevent impairment by managing our multiple reserve factors to enhance cognitive function and decrease the risk of age-related disease, as we'll see in the coming chapters.

PART II

APPLICATIONS: WHAT CAN WE DO ABOUT THE OPPORTUNITY OF AGING?

12 OVERVIEW

In the 1990s, I spoke at an Alzheimer's Association conference about my research on mental and physical activities
and disease risk. At a press conference, I suggested that
in order to lower the risk of Alzheimer's disease, people
should be physically and mentally active throughout life,
avoid smoking and obesity, eat a diet high in plant foods
and low in saturated fat, and properly manage diabetes
and hypertension. I explained how these recommendations were based on the work of my group as well as many
others from around the world.

When I concluded my remarks, an Alzheimer's Association official stood up, raised his arms out wide and said,
"Wait, Dr. Friedland's suggestions have not been verified
in a placebo-controlled, double-blind randomized trial,
and are premature."

I was dumbfounded. I responded by saying my recommendations were already known to be good for people
anyway, and that currently available research already suggested that they would be helpful. Also, people who follow
them (eat healthily, exercise, etc.) have no risk of side effects. It's true that some of the guidance recommendations
listed in the following chapters have not been comprehensively evaluated using double-blind, placebo-controlled,
randomized trials. It will be terrific when these studies are
completed, but we need to know what to do now. But not
everyone agrees with me.

In a 2010 "State-of-the-Science Conference statement:
preventing Alzheimer's disease and cognitive decline,"

researchers observed that diabetes, hyperlipidemia in midlife, and tobacco use were associated with an increased risk of Alzheimer's disease.[114] Mediterranean diet, folic acid intake, low or moderate alcohol intake, cognitive activities, and physical activities were associated with decreased risk. However, because the "quality of evidence was low for all of these associations" they were unable to draw firm conclusions on the association of any modifiable factors with the risk of Alzheimer's disease.[114,115]

In 2017, the US National Academies of Science, Engineering and Medicine led by Alan Leshner, CEO emeritus of the American Association for the Advancement of Science, and Story Landis, Director Emeritus of the National Institute of Neurological Disease and Stroke, also argued that the data were too weak to issue specific guidelines to the general public concerning what people can do to lower the risk of Alzheimer's disease.[116]

I strongly object to these conclusions. I met Shivani Nandi at a 1999 meeting of Alzheimer Disease International in Johannesburg, South Africa. We fell in love and married. Since we're both devoted to helping people avoid Alzheimer's disease, we collaborated on a paper published in 2013. Our satirical essay, "A modest proposal for a longitudinal study of dementia prevention (with apologies to Jonathan Swift, 1729)" in the *Journal of Alzheimer's Disease* focuses attention on the need for Alzheimer's disease prevention efforts.[34] We proposed a plan for a 40-year study of 10,000 people randomly assigned to groups of low- or high-saturated fat in the diet, head injury, high or low levels of mental and physical activity or inactivity, as well as smoking or non-smoking. Such a study is clearly impossible to conduct. Our point is that since this ideal study can't be accomplished, we must proceed with recommendations based on available evidence. It's simply not acceptable to wait for further information before recommendations can be made. Our "modest proposal" illustrates that the absence of definitive evidence should not restrict us from making reasonable recommendations based on the evidence that is already established. As the American astronomer and author Carl Sagan said, "The absence of evidence is not evidence of absence."

We know that hypertension and smoking are both risk factors for dementia. (We also know that they are risk factors for heart disease and stroke, as well as other conditions.) Why was it not recommended by the eminent panels that government and institutional bodies encourage better management of hypertension and avoidance of smoking in order to lower the dementia risk? What is the possible danger of such a recommendation? It has been estimated that risk factor reductions (similar to the ones I am recommending to you) could diminish the prevalence of Alzheimer's disease by 10 percent worldwide and 25 percent in the United States. About half of all Alzheimer's cases are thought to be potentially attributable to hypertension and smoking.

A recent analysis of 153 randomized clinical trials suggests the following factors may increase the risk of Alzheimer's disease:[117]

- low levels of education,
- low levels of cognitive activity (mental stimulation),
- low levels of physical exercise,
- low intake of vitamin C,
- high blood homocysteine levels,
- depression,
- stress,
- diabetes,
- head trauma,
- hypertension in midlife,
- obesity in midlife,
- significant weight loss in late life,
- smoking,

- poor sleep,
- cerebrovascular disease,
- frailty, and
- atrial fibrillation.

Before we consider how to implement recommendations concerning these risk factors, we must consider carefully the context of aging. An important aspect of these risk/protective factor considerations is that they involve several conditions, not only Alzheimer's disease. Hypertension, midlife physical inactivity, midlife obesity, and smoking are all risk factors for Alzheimer's disease, but they are also risk factors for cardiovascular disease and stroke. These conditions are linked to Alzheimer's disease itself: persons with heart disease and cerebrovascular disease are at a greater risk of Alzheimer's disease because heart disease and stroke reduce a person's physical reserve capacity and make it more likely that dementia will appear in the early stages of degenerative disease. Heart disease and stroke accelerate the Alzheimer's process in the brain. Red meat and low fiber intake are both risk factors for colon cancer. It is wise for me to offer these recommendations, and for you to heed them, because they are clearly beneficial to human health. Four factors are critical.

1. **Risk and protective factors operate over a lifetime.** With Carol Brayne of the University of Cambridge, I addressed these issues in a paper titled, "What does the pediatrician need to know about Alzheimer's disease?"[118] Early-life cognitive enrichment is associated with favorable cognitive health in late life, demonstrating clearly that preventive measures should be started as early as possible.[22] One main reason why there are no placebo-controlled, randomized trials to evaluate the influence of early-life factors is that they cannot be done; a clinical trial cannot be done over a 40-year period. Results of trials that show no benefit

over a three-year period do not mean that the intervention will not be effective if applied for a longer time.

The lifestyle factors reviewed in the following chapters apply to all phases of the life cycle, including the very early years. In a remarkable series of experiments, Michael Meaney and colleagues in Montreal have shown that maternal affection alters the packaging of genes in the hippocampus of baby rodents.[I] Animals who receive more maternal affection have more receptors on neurons in the hippocampus that are important for memory and learning.[119] They showed that animals receiving more maternal affection had a faster resolution of the stress response, improving survival of neurons and memory with aging. The beneficial effects of the mother's interaction with the baby have been assumed to be created through influences on the stress response. It may also be a result of the impact of the maternal contact on the baby's developing microbiota. There is a large literature showing that intimate contact between human mothers and babies is good for physical and psychological development.

The importance of children's exposure to microbes has been emphasized in a recent book from microbiota experts Jack Gilbert and Rob Knight. In their book *Dirt Is Good: The Advantage of Germs for Your Child's Developing Immune System*, they note that children who grow up with a dog have more competent immune systems than children who do not.[120]

2. **Alzheimer's disease takes several decades to develop and happens late in life. So our goal is not only to prevent it from developing, but also to delay its onset.** It is estimated that if the onset age of Alzheimer's disease can be delayed by five years the prevalence will be cut in

---

[I] This mechanism of gene alteration involves epigenetics, heritable changes in gene expression that do not involve changes to the DNA sequence.

half. By increasing the fitness of body systems which interact with the brain, as well as enhancing the fitness of the brain itself, we have the opportunity to alter disease processes over the course of a lifetime to delay the onset of dementia.[121]

3. **Environmental factors matter.** Recent studies have shown that the incidence and prevalence of Alzheimer's disease has dropped by about 20 percent in the past two decades (corrected for the fact that there are more older persons), according to studies in Europe, Asia, and the United States. A study of 1,599 older people found decreased markers of Alzheimer's pathology in the brain over a 30-year period.[122] This is almost certainly because of environmental factors: better education, medical care, living conditions, nutrition, control of hypertension and heart disease, and less smoking.[123] According to the US Census Bureau, among people aged 65 and older in 1965, only 5 percent had completed a bachelor's degree or more and, by 2018, this share had risen to 29 percent.[124] The observation that the risk of Alzheimer's disease is falling is strong support for the concept that preventive factors are important.

4. **Age does not need to limit our options.** Special problems may be encountered when encouraging older people to take preventive measures, as many older people and family members have rigid biases against the idea that they're capable of learning and of being physically active. A common view is that education applies only to the young. Many people also feel that if they are unable to run, they are unable to exercise. Furthermore, older persons often have less money than younger ones and have sensory deficits (visual, auditory, and vestibular), which impairs their opportunity to participate. They commonly have less access to transportation than the young. It is important to take these factors into account when planning lifestyle changes. Older persons can still exercise even if they can't

run. And alternate means of transportation may be needed for persons who can no longer drive.

Chapters 13 to 25 below provide a comprehensive discussion of lifestyle factors that may be considered in order to lower the risk of developing neurodegenerative disease, improve the body's resilience so that function can be maintained despite the development of disease, and enhance the capacity of the four reserve factors: cognitive, physical, psychological, and social. Enhancing these four reserve factors will enable you to augment your enjoyment of the opportunity that aging presents.

Enhancing these four reserve factors will enable you to augment your enjoyment of the opportunity that aging presents.

Changes in lifestyle behaviors, medications, and supplements should be discussed with a physician. I am not specific concerning the amount of exercise, dose of supplements, or targets for dietary consumption, because these figures will be highly variable from person to person and should be considered upon consultation with a physician.

13 PHYSICAL ACTIVITY

We don't stop playing because we grow old. We grow old because we stop playing.
George Bernard Shaw (1856–1950), Irish playwright and critic

When I was 30 years old, a 72-year-old cousin of mine had a heart attack. He was significantly overweight and did not exercise. Following the event, he embarked on a dietary and exercise program. I was glad that he was showing an appropriate response to his illness, but I thought how much better it would have been if he had started paying attention to his weight and lack of exercise 40 years earlier. This led me to consider my own dearth of physical activity. I played softball with a group of colleagues from the Lawrence Berkeley Laboratory. Our team was called the "Heavy Ions." The name for an opponent's team was the "Nads," because of the word that would result if their fans encouraged them to "Go … !" I felt that being on the softball team had a negative influence on my physical fitness, because I played right field and the ball was rarely hit in that direction. Also, after every game we went out drinking, and my beer consumption was considerable.

Shortly after my cousin's heart attack, I quit softball and began playing tennis. Although I'd previously played tennis, I did it sparingly and had only had seven lessons. I had no idea how to serve. I joined a tennis club, bought a new racket, and rationalized the expenses by asserting that the annual cost of my tennis hobby may be less than one or two ski trips, not counting the cost of knee surgeries from skiing accidents. My cousin died shortly thereafter. Over the past 40-plus years, I've continued to play tennis a few times a week throughout the year. Although I'm still struggling to serve and hit a backhand, I really love to play – it has helped me both physically and mentally. Tennis provides me with a form of intense mental concentration, which is valuable in relieving stress and enhancing my ability to focus attention.

We are not prepared by our genes for a sedentary lifestyle.

We are not prepared by our genes for a sedentary lifestyle. Studies have shown that higher levels of physical activity throughout life have beneficial effects on the development of Alzheimer's disease, as well as stroke, cardiovascular disease, and depression (in both humans and animals). Surprisingly, physical activity increases the production of new neurons in the brain that activates learning.

In addition, physical activity enhances the production of growth factors in the brain and in the liver, which can facilitate communication among neurons and the maintenance of mental function. These growth factors enhance the production and function of new neurons and aid the reliability of the brain's blood vessels. Exercise also enhances the immune system, producing more protective cells and antibodies, and assists with skeletal, endocrine, and cardiac health. The function of blood vessels in the heart, brain, and everywhere in the body is enhanced with exercise. Physical activity may also alleviate the effects of depression.

It is critical to recognize that most people are capable of some level of physical exercise: people who cannot run should walk, people who cannot walk comfortably should consider aquatherapy, where they can walk comfortably in a pool. Swimming is also terrific exercise. Our research has shown that people who become less physically and mentally active in the years from midlife to later life have a higher risk of developing Alzheimer's disease, compared to those whose participation stayed the same or became more active.[17]

Exercise has positive effects on all organ systems in the body.

Exercise has positive effects on all organ systems in the body. Moderate to vigorous exercise improves mental processing speed, memory and executive function, and sleep, and it may reduce or prevent depression. This is also true for both older and younger persons and persons with dementia. A Mayo Clinic study of over 2,000 people found that even light-intensity midlife physical activity decreased the decline in memory function with age.[125] Persons who are physically active for more than 150 minutes a week have a 33 percent lower risk of all-cause mortality than those who are sedentary. The beneficial effects of exercise of the brain are most marked in the hippocampus and prefrontal cortex, regions closely involved in cognitive function. Higher levels of physical activity have also been associated with increased cortical thickness. A study of over 16,000 Europeans and research from Australia found that regular exercise may improve brain function and diminish dementia risk.[7]

Critically, physical activity must not be dependent upon the weather. Many people go for a walk on beautiful days, but if it's raining or cold, they stay home. *If it's raining, the need for physical activity doesn't disappear!* Use home exercise equipment, join a gym, or go to a mall or other locations for a walk. Owning an exercise bike doesn't count as exercise if it isn't used.

Diversity is also an important goal for physical activity. Aerobic exercise is valuable for the heart, lungs, and the circulation. Strength training increases muscle mass and fortifies bones and joints. Stretching may also be helpful. All of these forms of exercise have beneficial effects on the brain. The deep breathing associated with exercise is beneficial for the lungs and heart.

The United States Department of Health and Human Services reports that less than 5 percent of adults in the United States engage in 30 minutes of physical activity each day, with only one in three adults attaining the suggested levels. Aerobic activities of 20–60 minutes, three to five times a week, and strength training, two to three times a week, are recommended.

Evidence shows that a lack of exposure to nature is an important factor in poor health and depression.

It's important to exercise in nature. Evidence shows that a lack of exposure to nature is an important factor in poor health and depression. Entomologist Edward Wilson of Harvard University has described the impact of our evolutionary history on our need for natural environments in his book *Biophilia* (biophilia means "love of life").[126] For most of the past 100,000 years of human history, our ancestors lived in close contact with the environment, and the ability to pay attention to the natural world was critical to their survival. Because of this, our brains have evolved the capacity for an appreciation and awareness of nature that is an essential feature of ourselves. Only in the last 100 years have many urbanites lived with limited contact with nature. Evidence for the importance of interaction with the biological world is substantial. For example, outdoor activities have been found to be more effective than antipsychotics for managing physical aggression in dementia.[108] It's also been reported that exposure to green vegetation can offset the negative effects of air pollution on the body's circulation.

It is good to be physically active throughout life. Walk instead of using elevators or escalators. When shopping, park farther away from the store to increase activity. Get exercise bands to use for stretching and strengthening while you watch movies at home. Understand that money spent on exercise is well spent. Better to spend money on a gym than on the hospitalization you may avoid by exercising. Watch out for talking yourself out of doing exercise: "I'll do it tomorrow"; "I'm tired"; "I did it yesterday"; "It's too cold"; "It's too hot"; "I can't do it right"; "I can't do it like I used to."

Many people do not exercise because of pain. It is certainly advisable to not do things that hurt. But it is best for you to find out what you can do without pain. Fifteen years ago, I had surgery on my left ankle and could not run, walk fast, play tennis, or use a treadmill. But I could use an exercise bike, which allowed me to continue exercising.

As we have discussed, exercise is important at every stage of life. Children need physical activity for proper growth of bones, joints, and muscles. Consider what children will do with the lifetime habits they develop in their early years. Few people play American football after the age of 20, and basketball is also largely a game for young people. I had to stop playing basketball at the age of 30 because of the multiple ankle injuries I sustained. Similarly, soccer, referred to as football in Europe, is challenging for people to play in midlife. It is therefore important for children to participate in a wide range of sports – including some that do not have a high rate of injuries – so they can continue playing those sports as they age. Tennis, golf, badminton, running, dance, martial arts, and swimming are certainly wonderful activities for children to learn to appreciate in their early years.

Why not try an experiment? For one month, engage in vigorous physical exercise every day (the duration and intensity of the exercise depends on many things, and you may choose to review with your doctor, of course). After this period, see if you feel better or worse. You may surprise yourself!

There are two chief rules of physical exercise that must be followed: (1) start; and (2) continue.

Physical exercise enhances all the four reserve factors.

Physical exercise enhances all the four reserve factors. It is good for the brain, all parts of the body, our mental attitude, and our social contacts.

14 WHOLE BODY HEALTH

The word systemic means pertaining to an entire organism. A critical component of the theory of the multiple reserve factors is that the health of the body is good for the health of the brain. The brain is dependent on all other body parts for the maintenance of its functions. This dependence of the brain upon other bodily functions is especially prominent in older persons, because of their lower reserve capacity. Research trials have shown that intensive blood pressure control (less than 120/80 mmHg) is more effective than standard blood pressure control (less than 140/90 mmHg) in reducing the risk of cognitive impairment.[61] It is certainly true that "what is good for the heart is good for the brain." It is also valuable to have the best possible heart, lung, kidney, liver, and endocrine function. Diabetes increases the risk of Alzheimer's disease as well as small and large strokes. It is related to diet, physical exercise, and obesity. A high-fiber diet can improve insulin responsiveness and diminish the severity of diabetes mellitus type 2. Many of the recommendations in this book are good for the health of the systemic health as well as directly beneficial to the nervous system. The word systemic means pertaining to an entire organism.

The brain is dependent on all other body parts for the maintenance of its functions.

Excess weight should be avoided. Obesity is a good example of the interactions amongst the four reserves. It is obvious that obesity can interfere with physical activity such as running. But the influence of obesity on neuro-degeneration, stroke, heart disease, and other conditions is more opaque. Obesity may reduce insulin responsiveness, cause diabetes, affect kidney and cardiac function, decrease the effectiveness of the immune system, damage gut bacteria, accelerate vascular disease, increase the risk of colon cancer, and contribute to the development of strokes. Obesity has been linked to the presence of gut bacteria that are more efficient in "harvesting" nutrition from the diet. A high-fiber diet may help avoid obesity (see Chapter 20).

To maintain good physical reserve, it is important to do what you can to avoid toxic exposures, at home and at work (discussed in Chapter 25). Be aware of the fact that toxic factors can impair your reserve capacity without making you sick. That is, your fitness may be reduced without any symptoms or signs. As I have shown, in order to be able to enjoy the opportunity of aging, we need to have the best possible reserve capacity so that we can respond well to challenges that develop.

Good systemic health means good physical reserve. Good physical reserve helps to maintain healthy brain function throughout life.

15 MENTAL ACTIVITY

As noted in an earlier chapter, a series of 1980s research studies showed a strong relationship between the prevalence and incidence of Alzheimer's disease and years spent in education.[127] According to the studies, people with more years of education had a lower risk of developing the disease.

Television and Aging

Americans love television, certainly too much. In 2015, US viewers watched about three hours per day, more than people in any other country. Television viewing is a uniquely passive experience. Not only does it not allow participation, but it also actively discourages participation. While it is possible to be involved in learning while watching television, educational programs are not the most widespread viewing activity. Most television programs don't require much intellectual activity. Think about what happens when you are reading a book: the pages do not turn if you fall asleep. To read a book you must participate. And if you have a question about what's happening in the book, you can go back and read a previous page. This is generally impossible while watching television. Evidence shows that sedentary activities such as television viewing increase the risk of heart disease, cancer, and death, with dose-dependent associations – on the other hand, studies report that reading can reduce your risk of cognitive decline in later life, no matter how much education you've had.

A Korean study of 9,644 people found that television viewing was a significant risk factor of cognitive dysfunction, along with a lack of participation in physical activities.[128] It is likely that television viewing is a marker for a mentally inactive state. Longer television viewing times have also been significantly associated with the risk of cardiovascular disease.[129,130] A sedentary lifestyle is also associated with frailty, and it has been shown that reading and physical exercise may prevent frailty in older persons with mild cognitive impairment.[131]

Learning Is the Work of the Brain

A life filled with learning is certainly advisable. Tasks involving some degree of cognitive complexity is desirable, but there is no reason to believe that certain forms of learning are better than others. What is critical here is that the activity needs to be consistent and persistent. Involvement of cognitive activity at work is important and jobs that involve high stress, passive participation, and lack of complexity are associated with higher levels of cognitive impairment in later life.

People are able to learn at all ages and participation in learning is valuable for the brain throughout life.

There is also absolutely no reason to believe that mental activities must be limited to the early years of life. People are able to learn at all ages and participation in learning is valuable for the brain throughout life. I have often been asked what form of mental activity is best for the brain. While there is no definitive evidence to inform the best answer to this question, it is clear that activities that involve learning are best.

Because of my interest in enhancing opportunities for cognitively stimulating activities, I helped create the Checkmating Dementia Foundation, to encourage people to play chess. Playing chess involves anticipating future situations and analyzing possible outcomes. It also involves interactions with at least one other person, is inexpensive, and can be played on the internet. The development of the foundation has been slow, perhaps because many people have never learned how to play. I learned to play as a child but have never developed an understanding of chess strategy. I taught my son to play chess as a boy and remember the days when I could beat him. That was when he was about 11. But soon after that he said he didn't like playing me anymore because he beat me too easily. (Who can blame him?) At the Checkmating Dementia Foundation, we're hoping to encourage people of all ages to play cognitively enhancing games.

Musical activities are valuable. Musical performance has important physical components. Listening to music often involves social interactions and provides relief from stress. Occupational activities are also important. Our research showed that people with Alzheimer's disease were more likely than healthy controls to have had jobs that were not mentally stimulating.[132] Working at a job that requires high levels of mental activity may be protective against dementia in late life. Many other factors are at play here as well, as all these risk factors are more prevalent in people who have low levels of mental stimulation at work: toxic exposures, stress, poverty, poor access to healthcare, less education, and work injuries.

The concept of diversity refers as well to learning and mental activities. It is good to learn new things! Participation in cognitive activities throughout the lifespan, both at home and at work, can help build our cognitive reserve capacity. Furthermore, cognitive activities directly impair the disease process itself. Being cognitively active helps to protect the brain from free radicals and toxins. Cognitive activities also assist in the management of stress.

Choosing activities that involve learning should be fun. If you don't enjoy the activity, you will not do it. Don't allow yourself to be intimidated by the task at hand. What is important is the involvement of your brain and your enjoyment and appreciation of learning. Recognize the importance of small goals. For example, if you decide to take up watercolor painting, don't expect to be exhibited at a local museum. At least not until you have more experience!

Attention, Forgetting, and Distraction

William James wrote the following in his book *Principles of Psychology* (first published in 1890) (the emphasis is mine):

Millions of items of the outward order are present to my senses which never properly enter into my experience. Why? Because they have no interest for me. My experience is what I agree to attend to. *Only those items which I notice shape my mind-without selective interest, experience is an utter chaos. Interest alone gives accent and emphasis, light and shade, background and foreground-intelligible perspective, in a word. It varies in every creature, but without it, the consciousness of every creature would be a gray chaotic indiscriminativeness, impossible for us even to conceive.*

William James' words illustrate the vital distinction between experience (what happens to you) and attention (what you do with what happens to you).

The three components of memory – encoding, storage, and retrieval – are all necessary for a memory of an event to take place. Memory can fail when attention does not allow proper processing. If the memory is not properly stored there may be failure to recall. Retrieval may fail following the proper encoding and storage of a memory if it cannot be found. Frequently, retrieval fails in older persons when words which are well known cannot be located. This situation, often called "tip-of-the-tongue phenomenon," is, by definition, a sign of poor retrieval, but it can also be because of poor encoding or poor storage. A key strategy to improve memory is to devote more attention to an event which will assist in embedding the event in your memory. Proper analysis of the event makes storage more salient. Retrieval is better when encoding and storage have been well completed.

A key strategy to improve memory is to devote more attention to an event which will assist in embedding the event in your memory.

The focusing of attention can have a profound effect on memory. Older people have a reduced capacity for doing two things at once. Despite the enormous complexity of the brain, even at young ages we cannot do two cognitive tasks at the same time as effectively as we could accomplish them independently. Hearing in older persons is more sensitive to interference produced by ambient noise. It is advisable to find comfortably quiet surroundings whenever possible. Many restaurants and other social gathering places play loud music and have poor acoustics design, making it difficult for older people to hear conversations and to pay appropriate attention – making it all the easier to forget what's been said at all. It might be necessary to avoid these places.

One excellent way to improve memory is through stories.

Humans have evolved a tremendous capacity to appreciate and process stories. One excellent way to improve memory is through stories. For most of human history, stories were the main method by which information was transferred. Only in the twentieth century did a large proportion of persons became literate – before this, stories were memories passed down from generation to generation, verbally. Keeping history alive meant it was vital for humans to remember tales told, in order to pass them on. Our brains evolved in an environment where stories were treasured and the attention to stories was often the difference between life and death. Paying attention to what happens to you helps to make stories of what happens, which enhances memory.

Despite big changes in society and technology, we still have the same neurological capacities as our ancestors and still have a profound innate appreciation for stories. Our memory is enhanced whenever we can encode our memories as stories. When you learn, work on putting your new information in context. If you are watching a video on Queen Mary I of England (also known as Bloody Mary), take the time to read about her and her father, Henry VIII. If you enjoy walking in a local park, read about its history. When you meet new people, learn about them (discover what their story is). This requires both attention and understanding.

16 PSYCHOLOGICAL MEASURES

If you believe that feeling bad or worrying long enough will change a past or future event, then you are residing on another planet with a different reality system.

William James (1842–1910), American philosopher and psychologist

Management of Our Psychological Reserve Factor

It is necessary to maintain healthy and productive responses to the stresses and declines associated with aging. A key factor is the choice of attitude. Is the glass half empty or is it half full? Or do we have the wrong glass? It is critical for people to see opportunities for growth in aging – they are there to be had.

It is critical for people to see opportunities for growth in aging – they are there to be had.

As we discussed in Chapter 3, aging is accompanied by declines in the speed of learning, working memory, and memory capacity. These changes are found in nearly everyone. Many measures can be considered to help deal with this matter. The first approach is to realize that these declines are not caused by disease and are nearly universal. An older person may take longer to absorb the complex plots in a nineteenth-century Russian novel, but reading such a work is not a time-based competition and is to be encouraged. For the most part, small changes in cognition do not significantly impact occupational or social activities.

There are some limits, of course. It's certainly not wise for an 80-year-old person to take up air traffic control as a new endeavor. The multitasking involved and the need for instant life-and-death decisions suggest it would be better left for younger persons. But an 80-year-old person may indeed learn a new language, begin piano lessons, explore the waterfalls of Croatia (in person or online), study the genealogy of their family, or countless other beneficial undertakings.

It's important to recognize that the cognitive and memory capacities of older people aren't as good as those of the young. So, devoting memory resources to what is important, and ignoring things that are not important, is an excellent strategy. Keeping lists can help lessen the need to remember things to do.

Memory strategies may also help considerably. Instead of flinging your keys down anywhere when you get home, leave them in the same place every time – it will be easier to remember where they are when you need them. If you are aware in the evening that you will need an umbrella the following day, consider putting the umbrella on the door so when you leave the next day you will be certain to notice it. Forgetfulness is often linked to inattention, as noted by Ralph Waldo Emerson, American essayist and philosopher, who said, "It is found that we remember best when the head is clear, when we are thoroughly awake."

I recommend a book by Andrew E. Budson and Maureen K. O'Connor on this topic, *Seven Steps to Managing Your Memory: What's Normal, What's Not, and What to Do About It,* which contains valuable advice about ways to help your memory.[133]

A goal for healthy living is acceptance of life events and the appreciation of each new day.

A goal for healthy living is acceptance of life events and the appreciation of each new day. If anger, resentment, regret, and disappointment is carried over from month to month and year to year, the negative influence on the quality of life with aging can be substantial. As Gautama Buddha said, "Holding on to anger is like grasping a hot coal with the intent of throwing it at someone else; you are the one who gets burned."

Healthy aging involves the understanding that there are things that can't be changed and must be accepted. This does not mean that these stressful life events must be forgotten. Hopefully, they can be remembered with progressively less pain. The best way to avoid negative emotions caused by events and experiences in the past is to be actively involved in the present moment and planning for the future. Meditation is a valuable method to practice letting go and enhancing your awareness of the opportunities that are available now.[134]

The best way to avoid negative emotions caused by events and experiences in the past is to be actively involved in the present moment and planning for the future.

Aging also presents an opportunity to demonstrate self-compassion. As Buddhist teacher Cheri Huber said, "Joy is compassion turned inward." Frequently, persons express compassion to others throughout their lives with loving devotion and selfless actions, without realizing that that are worthy of compassion themselves.

The Search for Meaning

William James speculated that: "The deepest principle of human nature is the craving to be appreciated."[135] It is wise to define for yourself what is it that gives your life meaning. The psychiatrist Viktor Frankl demonstrated that the search for meaning was a key factor in human activities. "Those who have a 'why' to live can bear with almost any how," he said.

It is wise to define for yourself what is it that gives your life meaning.

Meaning is often lost as friends and family members die, jobs disappear, and activity is impaired by illness, disability, and lack of money. It is critical that we hold on to our uniqueness, and pursue meaning through work, hobbies, relationships, and activities. There are no right or wrong answers in the search for meaning, it is something that everyone must do for themselves. Viktor Frankl's book, *Man's Search for Meaning*, is an excellent place to start.[1]

At a music camp many years ago, I met an 82-year-old woman who was playing the viola da gamba, an instrument that was popular several hundred years ago, which is similar to the cello. The woman had been studying the viola de gamba for only a few years and was already playing in an orchestra. Because of my interest in cognitively stimulating activities, I asked if I could photograph her.

"Of course," she said, "Please take my picture and send it to me, I want it to show it to my grandchildren. I want them to see that I'm playing in a real orchestra."

At the end of the rehearsal, she put her instrument in a specially built backpack so she could rush to her next

---

[1]   *Man's Search for Meaning* was listed as "one of the ten most influential books in the US" by the Library of Congress in 1979.

class. Playing a musical instrument in an orchestra was something she had always wanted to do. She was able to accomplish this in her 70s and 80s, giving her great pride. Not only was learning a musical instrument a cognitive accomplishment, it also enhanced her self-confidence and self-worth, introduced her to other people, and provided physical activity.

It is wise not to wait until retirement to decide where to find meaning. At all stages of life, we should explore what are our unique interests and abilities and pursue them. It's common for people not to follow their interests in childhood because of financial matters or lack of family support. Middle and later ages provide an opportunity to renew previous interests. I have had patients with mild age-related changes who had played the piano earlier in life, and now rarely played. I gave them a signed order on my prescription pad, "Play the piano!"

Rabindranath Tagore wrote, "I slept and dreamt that life was joy. I awoke and saw that life was service. I acted and behold, service was joy." This statement by the Nobel Prize-winning Bengali poet confirms the view advanced by this book that meaning is a key to happiness and contentment.

Meditation

Some time every day devoted to silence and meditation may be of enormous value.

Meditation can be of great value in dealing with stress, anxiety, and depression. A recent study from Norway showed that mindfulness practice helps counter negative views of oneself and enhances self-reassurance.[136] Many people have busy lives and are rarely exposed to silence. Clearly, the brain needs time to adapt to changing situations and to regulate itself. Some time every day devoted to silence and meditation may be of enormous value. Silence is not required for mediation and in can be practiced while walking, gardening, or during many other activities. Negative thoughts may not be eliminated, but meditation can help obtain distance from the thoughts. There are many varieties of meditation including those from the traditions of Buddhism (mindfulness and Zen), Hinduism, Islam, Christianity, and Judaism. The Buddhist technique involves sitting comfortably in silence with the mind observing the body and the thoughts that arise. The task is not to stop thinking but rather to observe your own consciousness. It is best to find a comfortable sitting position with as little movement or muscle tension as possible. Hopefully, the only part of you that is moving is your breathing. When you stop moving, the body's sensations become quiet because of habituation. That is, when you put on your socks you can feel the socks going on your feet. But once they are on and the sensation is not changing, you can no longer feel them. As you remain still in meditation, the only thing you notice is what is moving – your breath and your mind. At the very least, such a practice is a rehearsal of "letting go." Meditative practice is best when performed daily. Meditation also lowers blood pressure and heart rate and improves the response to stress. There are many books that can assist people in learning meditation.[134]

Many people find activities such as fishing, walking in the woods, bird watching, swimming, and many others to be relaxing. I encourage you to find places that help to settle the mind. To quote William James once again, "Most people live in a very restricted circle of their potential being. They make use of a very small portion of their possible consciousness, and of their soul's resources in general, much like a man who, out of his whole organism should get into a habit of using and moving only his little finger."

Denial

No one wants to be sick. But denying illness can be dangerous. During a check-up, I asked one of my elderly patients,
a woman with severe dementia with disorientation, what
year it was. "Nineteen forty-two," she answered.

No one wants to be sick. But denying illness can
be dangerous.

Her adult daughter laughed. "Oh, she doesn't pay attention to current events," she said, implying that such a
great error was not significant. It is important to recognize
the cognitive bias we all have which may stop us appreciating the potential significance of a problem. That is, we
don't want to be sick and may not recognize evidence of
impairment in ourselves or others. This situation can extend from the patient having the difficulty to the family
and community. An extreme example of widespread denial happened during President Ronald Reagan's first term in
office. The president was displaying cognitive troubles. His
deficits were obvious, yet his condition was not properly
recognized by Reagan's associates, his doctors, or the general public. His Alzheimer's disease diagnosis wasn't made
public until 1994, a full five years after he left office.

People with brain disease can have deficits that they
might not be aware of and they may explicitly deny their
presence. A person with memory loss from Alzheimer's
disease might deny that there is any memory problem at
all – this may be because they don't remember their episodes of forgetting. It may also be a loss of insight into
the presence of the disability. Denial can also occur with
non-neurological illnesses and can often contribute to a
delayed diagnosis and improper management.

Denial may be explicit or implicit. A person may state
that there is nothing wrong and refuse to consider the

possibility when confronted with evidence (explicit denial). At times, people may demonstrate some awareness of a problem but are unwilling to make a reasonable effort to have it evaluated (implicit denial). Both forms of denial can lead to lack of recognition of illness, which can delay treatment.

Denial of cognitive deficit is a special problem because people may forget that they forgot and have poor comprehension because of the cognitive deficit. This form of denial is often shared with the family who might say, "Oh, she's 82 years old, what do you expect?" or "Well, there's nothing you can do about it anyway." Both of these approaches are dangerous and improper.

Significant cognitive impairment with or without dementia is not normal at any age. A 95-year-old person who is demonstrating significant memory loss should receive a medical evaluation because it's possible the condition is treatable and reversible (see Chapter 7). The management of this situation may significantly improve the quality of that person's life (see Case Study 9). Many people suspected of having Alzheimer's disease, including later ages, actually have a different problem that can be resolved if detected by a physician in time.

There is also, of course, denial of risk factors. Heavy drinkers may deny their alcoholism. Obese people may deny their condition. Similar considerations apply to smoking, high-fat diets, lack of exercise, and failure to seek medical care. People who deny an illness may fail to take their medications or comply with medical advice.

Denial may also involve reluctance or inability to change lifestyle actions (denial of the ability to change). "I am too old to exercise" is one example and "I haven't gone bowling in 40 years" is another. It is valuable to consider the risk–benefit ratio. Try one month of daily exercise for at least 30 minutes a day and see if it has a positive effect. What is the risk?

Case Study 9

A 71-year-old man came into my office with a complaint from his wife that he had memory impairment. An MRI scan revealed a normal amount of atrophy of the brain. Mental status testing showed that his memory and word-finding abilities were preserved and his scores on cognitive evaluation tests were good. He was an avid golfer and knew the rules of the game and recent events in the sport.

He was significantly overweight. At 5 foot 6 inches, he weighed 215 pounds and had a body mass index (BMI) of 34. (In the United States, a BMI score of 20–24 is normal, 25–29 is overweight, and 30 or more is obese.) He had moderate hypertension, didn't exercise, and ate a diet high in saturated fat. He hadn't seen a dentist in several years and drank two beers and one cocktail every night. While his memory was normal at this time, I encouraged him to exercise more and drink less. He didn't really believe he had a problem, explaining he once weighed 240 pounds and previously drank four to six beers a day. He wrapped up his philosophy to life this way: "When you're gonna go, you're gonna go."

I gently asked him if he looked both ways before crossing the street. If he did look, perhaps he wasn't really as ready to go as he thought. I wished to challenge him to confront the choices he was making.

Despite his reluctance, I reviewed the importance of improving his diet and exercise. I told him that many 71-year-old men will not live to be age 80, and that his chance of living longer will be substantially improved if he changed his lifestyle. He told me he wasn't afraid of dying. I explained that the situation was more complicated, since most people do not get to choose how or when they die. He could have a stroke and live another 20 years, paralyzed and mute.

I also suggested he take better care of his teeth and told him that good oral health is good for the brain and heart, as well as the teeth. We discussed the fact that his liver was 71 years old and may no longer be able to metabolize alcohol at the amount he is drinking, which can have serious consequences for his health. I also explained that the chance of him being able to continue playing golf when he was 80 would be significantly improved if he altered his lifestyle. I learned that he was very fond of his granddaughter who was 12 years of age. I asked if he wanted to be there when she graduated from high school. Did he want her to have her high-school graduation saddened by the fact that her grandfather was not there? And I explained that he may very well shortly be unable to play golf because of heart disease and diabetes.

Such denial of personal responsibility is an enormous problem. If it could be measured properly it may be one of the five leading causes of death. It is often a struggle to appreciate that what we do with our lives makes a difference. I hope the perspective provided by the concept of the opportunity of aging outlined in this book will help.

17 SOCIAL FACTORS

Man is by nature a social animal.
Aristotle (384–322 BCE), Greek philosopher

Humans are social beings and relationships with family, friends, and colleagues are critical for health at all stages of life. Studies have shown a higher risk of dementia in later life in individuals with poor social interactions. At all stages of life, it's desirable for people to have healthy relationships with others. Maintaining a socially active lifestyle in later life enhances cognitive reserve and benefits cognitive function.[25] The physical component of social interactions is also of value. Interpersonal experiences can influence the structure and function of the brain in both early and later life.[127] Opportunities for interactions with other people enhance social reserve and improve cognitive, physical, and psychological reserves.

Opportunities for interactions with other people enhance social reserve and improve cognitive, physical, and psychological reserves.

Studies of the relationship of social contacts to cognitive loss with aging suggest that dementia is more common in those whose social engagement declines from midlife to late life. It may be that declining social participation is caused by the development of cognitive losses. It is undoubtedly true that having stronger social contacts protects people from the manifestations of impairment that is a critical matter in age-related conditions.

Social interactions have always been important to humans. Even in the twenty-first century, we need close contact with others. We need to care for others, and we need to be cared for. Physical contact, like giving hugs, has important beneficial influence on our feeling state as well as on our endocrine system, stress responses, and blood pressure. People in long-term relationships are at lower risk of getting dementia. Social contacts increase physical activity that may improve the stress response and improve heart health. I may decide that I need to exercise on a certain day but decide that I am too tired and stay home. If I then get a call from a friend asking to go and play tennis, I may very well go, as I love to play and I know that my friend may be unable to play without me. Thereby social factors are enhancing my physical activity.

It is critical to develop supportive and durable social networks throughout life. Even at advanced ages it is necessary to look for opportunities to connect with others (as noted in Amanda Barusch's *Love Stories of Later Life*).[137] The loss of social contacts with aging because of the death of family members and friends, sensory and physical impairment, and lack of funds is an enormous problem for older people around the world.

Pets can help expand social interactions for people of all ages. Dog ownership is associated with lower blood pressure, better lipid profiles, and improved responses to stress. A systematic review of studies from 1950 to 2019 shows that owning a dog was accompanied by a 25 percent reduction in mortality (compared to non-ownership) and a 30 percent reduction in death from heart disease. Dog ownership is also associated with better physical and cognitive function because, of course, owners need to walk their golden retrievers and regal French bulldogs. I have often found that people who live in my neighborhood do not stop to talk to each other. A dog is an excellent factor to initiate conversation between strangers.

An aunt of mine at the age of 80 traveled alone to England. In London, she stayed at a bed and breakfast and went down one day for the morning meal. She was seated at a lovely table by the garden. The concierge came and asked if she would mind if a certain gentleman joined her table, because they were quite full that day and there were no available seats. My aunt said that she would be delighted and was surprised to see that the man who was joining her lived in her apartment building in Manhattan. They had seen each other in the elevator for more than 10 years but had unfortunately never spoken. Now that they were sharing a table in a London guesthouse, they found that they had many things in common and they became friends. The man took my aunt out for dinner one night a month for over 10 years. It is my experience that while traveling you often meet people in very novel and mysterious ways.

Social interactions can be enhanced in aging through community organizations, social action groups, religious activities, and travel. Pursuing activities that help you find meaning will also help you make social connections.

18 DEALING WITH STRESS

From the point of view of human evolution, it's important to remember critical things that happen to us. If, 10,000 years ago, an ancestor of ours walked to a river to get water and saw an attractive bird, she might or might not have remembered that event. But if she was attacked by a crocodile and managed to barely escape, she'd definitely have remembered that. Such an event is of adaptive value to remember. That is, remembering the event might have saved her life another day (the memory might have helped her to not go to the place of the attack and to watch carefully for crocodiles). Also, she would likely have told the story to others. Remembering the event is critical. And it is evolutionarily advantageous for her to remember it, unlike the memory of the bird.

During stress, the endocrine and brain systems involved have distinct neurochemical processes which enhance the salience (power) of the memory. The tenacious nature of post-traumatic stress disorder (PTSD) is due not only to psychological factors, but neurochemical and evolutionary ones as well. It is valuable for people who have experienced stressful life events to realize that the power these memories have is not entirely psychological. Rather, it is in a deeply developed neural pathway created and preserved in the brain in a resilient fashion. Understanding that this is not a question primarily of "getting over it," but rather "learning to live with it" may help.

Stress has many effects on the brain and the body. It is clear that bolstering your physical reserves with physical activity, effective sleep, and a healthy diet enhances the ability to deal with stress. The experience of stress involves not only the brain, but also the body's cardiovascular system and other parts.

It is difficult to measure stress in humans, as people respond to stress differently (what is stressful for one person may be a joy to another). In the stress response, there are pathways of neural and endocrine systems that enhance the person's ability to act during an emergency. The adrenal hormones (called glucocorticoids, such as cortisol) influence the heart as well as the brain. These responses are adaptive in stressful situations, but not normal, everyday situations. Considerable research suggests that a critical factor is how quickly the stress response recovers. Animal and human studies show that babies who received relatively more maternal affection have better stress responses in later life, as well as increased survival of neurons with age. These effects may be related to changes in the adaptability of the stress response, as well as different exposures to the mother's microbiota. Stress can be a critical aspect of complex cognitive tasks that are enjoyed by some people. For others, the stressful aspect of those same tasks may be unpleasant. If an activity is so stressful that it inhibits participation, it is clearly not beneficial to health.

Studies show that a history of stress-related conditions increases the risk of vascular cognitive impairment or Alzheimer's disease. This includes PTSD, acute stress reactions, and adjustment disorders. A recent analysis of many studies shows PTSD is especially threatening to human health, perhaps doubling the risk of dementia from all causes in late life.[138] Individuals who suffer stressful life events may develop behavioral and functional problems later in life because of the reduced capacity of the brain to maintain adaptation to the stress. It is best if the work of dealing with stressful factors is accomplished as quickly as possible, before the achievement of great age.

Studies show that a history of stress-related conditions increases the risk of vascular cognitive impairment or Alzheimer's disease.

Several strategies can help to deal with stress: restful sleep, meditation, a healthy diet, cognitive and physical exercise, social interactions, counseling and psychotherapy, and the avoidance of toxins (alcohol, smoking) and polypharmacy (incorrect use of drugs). It is important to understand that often stress is not the problem – the problem is our response to the stress.

19 SLEEP

Sleep is incredibly important for the creation and maintenance of memories. It is an active process managed by the brain to allow for bodily rest and the repair and maintenance of homeostasis. Good sleep is necessary for life and health and is essential for the encoding and storage of memories made during wakefulness. Poor sleep can interfere with all aspects of cognitive function, particularly attention and memory and has been linked to depression and impaired immune function. The length (amount) of sleep is not the only important factor; the quality of sleep is also vital. Animal studies have revealed that sleep deprivation damages gut bacteria and produces hazardous free radicals, called oxidative stress.

Cognitive reserve is closely related to sleep. Too many people take sleep for granted or think getting a restful sleep is a luxury, not a necessity. But recent research shows the pattern of neuronal firing is replayed during sleep, which enhances the formation of memories.

As we age, sleeping problems often become more frequent and may impact the quality of life.

Sleep disturbances are seen in several neurodegenerative diseases and are among the earliest symptoms of Alzheimer's disease, including reduced total, slow wave, and rapid eye movement (REM) sleep time. This is worrisome and potentially dangerous because sleep impairments can accelerate Alzheimer's pathology in the brain and increase the risk of Alzheimer's disease, dementia, and stroke.[139]

Research has also shown how sleep deprivation increases Alzheimer's-related proteins in humans and rodents.

People with Parkinson's disease or Lewy body disease may have excessive movements during sleep, including violent ones. This is called rapid eye movement behavioral sleep disorder and may develop even before the motor or cognitive signs of these disorders. This sleep problem can often be well managed with medications.

Recently, it's been discovered that sleep influences the clearance of the Alzheimer's-related neuronal proteins in the brain. During sleep it is believed that a network of pathways along blood vessels is active in clearing potentially toxic substances from the brain. This pathway is particularly active during sleep. The many short- and long-term negative influences of lack of sleep may be related to impaired clearance of toxic molecules from the brain. Research has shown that short afternoon naps (10 to 20 minutes) reduce the risk of five-year cognitive decline in older persons.

There are many things one can do to improve the quality of sleep:

- Go to sleep at the same time every night.
- The bed and bedroom should be used only for sleep and amorous activity, and not for other tasks, such as watching television, texting friends, reading Facebook, or paying bills.
- Don't sleep with your phone on or place it near your bed. Put it in another room and turn the ringer off.
- Watching the news just before bedtime may lead to anxiety and poor sleep. It's unlikely that you will see a story on the news such as "We're very happy tonight to report that Pakistan and India have decided to cease hostilities and open their borders." That would be wonderful! But unfortunately, it's more likely that you will hear on the news about a disaster or murder that may consciously or unconsciously disturb your sleep.

- Don't drink caffeinated beverages after 4 p.m.
- Melatonin taken at bedtime may help initiate sleep and may also enhance memory, according to some studies (it is also an antioxidant).
- Drink less water during the evening if you have a problem with frequent urination at night.
- Keep the bedroom relatively cool and have the room as dark and quiet as possible.
- If you don't fall asleep within 20 minutes, get up and go to another room and sit on a chair. Try not to associate the anxiety of not sleeping with your bed.
- If you have episodes of arrested breathing during sleep (apnea) or snoring, ask your doctor for a sleep study (polysomnogram) referral.
- If your sleep is interrupted by anxiety and depression, seek help from a counselor, psychiatrist, psychologist, and possibly consider antidepressant medication.
- If you're over 65 years of age, avoid using antihistamines for sleep (this includes Tylenol PM and a wide range of other medications listed in Chapter 23).
- If you regularly take naps and have problems sleeping at night, limit or stop napping during the day.
- Do not try to sleep, as sleep cannot be achieved on command. It is a natural process which occurs spontaneously.
- Do not have physical exercise within three hours of bedtime.
- If you go to bed at 10 p.m. and find that you wake up at 1 or 2 a.m. and cannot get back to sleep, consider moving your sleep time back to 11 p.m. or midnight.
- When you are asleep, molecules made in the brain that may be dangerous are removed through pathways along blood vessels. This process may work better when you are not lying on your back so consider sleeping in another position.

20 DIET

Everything in moderation, including moderation.
Oscar Wilde (1854–1900), Irish playwright

Overview and Evolutionary Considerations

Our dietary choices affect our health and fitness in two ways. First, diet has a direct influence on the brain and other body parts – for example, a diet high in saturated fat accelerates vessel degeneration and leads to a higher risk of coronary artery disease and stroke. Second, dietary choices influence the nature of our microbial populations in the gut. These two mechanisms frequently work together; a high-salt diet can make high blood pressure worse and will influence the nature of the microbiota in the gut, increasing inflammation – two processes which increase the risk of heart disease and stroke.

The bottom line is: dietary choices determine what food is available for our microbiota, which influences what organisms are present. And the nature of our microbial communities has a profound influence on our health and fitness. Our dietary choices strongly affect our health through a direct influence on our organ systems.

Our ancestors had a diet quite different than the one we have today. Studies of hunter–gatherer communities around the world show that their diet had less saturated fat and much greater diversity and more fiber than most humans are eating now. The genes we have that keep us healthy were selected in the past because they were adaptive when our ancestors were consuming this earlier diet. Our genes did not develop in response to our current consumption patterns.

For example, beef has more than five times more fat than the meat eaten by our ancestors, which would have been meats such as deer. Nearly all beef consumed in the United States comes from grain-fed, factory-farmed cattle, with a higher content of harmful saturated fatty acids. Beef from grain-fed cattle has fewer of the beneficial omega-3 fatty acids and monounsaturated fatty acids than grass-fed cattle.

We also eat less seafood than our ancestors did. It's estimated that in the early modern human diet, up to 50 percent of energy consumption was from seafood. This provided them with n-3 fatty acids, particularly docosahexaenoic acid. This molecule is an important component of brain membranes and likely assisted in the evolution of our immune and nervous systems. Red meat has more saturated fat than chicken, fish, or vegetable protein sources such as beans. Red meat also contains more carcinogens and oxidants produced in cooking. A study of over 450,000 adults in the United Kingdom showed that consumption of red meat was associated with an increased risk of coronary artery disease, as well as pneumonia and diabetes.[140] Eating red and processed meat is associated with a higher risk of colorectal cancer, heart disease, and diabetes. (Avoid the burger please.)

Our ancestors had a varied diet because of the seasons, the influence of the weather, and the migration of animals and humans. Before the invention of salting and smoking, humans also had limited means to preserve food. Today, many people eat similar things for breakfast, lunch, and dinner, all year long. This was not possible in the past. Diversity of healthy foods is critical for diversity of the "good" microbiota, which are valuable for health and fitness: your physical reserve factor.

Diversity

The concept of diversity is a key element in this discussion. We need a diverse bacterial community for health. If our internal bacterial population is not diverse, we have an imbalance in gut bacteria, which leads to disease or dysfunction (digestive disturbances such as bloating, constipation, stomach cramps, amongst others). To foster the presence of complex bacterial communities, we need diverse diets that meet the nutritional requirements of many different kinds of bacteria.

We need a diverse bacterial community for health.

Fiber

Fiber is a component of complex carbohydrates that can't be digested by humans but is metabolized in the gut by bacteria that make molecules important for human health and help prevent disease. High-fiber foods include whole grains, fruit, vegetables, legumes, brown rice, and beans – but fiber is not found in meat. Beans are high in protein, fiber, minerals, vitamins, and antioxidants. Whole grains have vitamins, minerals, and other helpful compounds.

To support a diverse microbiome in the gut, eat a variety of fiber-rich food. One cup of cooked kidney beans has about 10 grams of fiber, which is a considerable amount. Legumes such as green beans, chickpeas, and lentils are also terrific because they are low in fat and high in nutritional value. They are high in protein, fiber, B vitamins, and minerals. Legumes lower cholesterol and blood pressure, assist weight control, and help people avoid diabetes.

There is no good reason to eat white bread. It has one-half of the fiber and less protein than whole wheat bread.

An analysis of 45 studies found that consumption of whole grains lowered the risk of heart disease and stroke, as well as death.[141]

It is currently recommended that people consume 35 grams of fiber a day. However, researchers have studied the diets of hunter–gatherer communities existing today and found that they consume much more fiber than this suggested consumption level, indicating that perhaps our target should be higher. The thought is that our ancestors were hunter–gatherers for much of the past 100,000 years, and that was the time during which our genes were selected. This suggests that our genetic inheritance is best prepared for a high-fiber diet. Fiber increases the production of regulatory immune cells that are effectively anti-inflammatory.[142] And fiber also helps keep the gut barrier strong in defending against bacterial invasion and improving metabolism.[143,144] A study of over 133,700 people in 21 countries found that a high intake of highly processed (refined) grains is associated with a higher risk of heart disease and death than unrefined (whole) grains.[145] Refined grains have been milled and are not whole, and are missing important parts of the plant, such as bran and germ. They have fewer vitamins and minerals than whole grains. Refined grains include white flour, white rice, corn grits, and white bread. Studies have shown that a higher whole-grain intake is associated with a lower risk of cardiovascular disease and death.

If you're concerned about celiac disease (also called celiac sprue or gluten-sensitive enteropathy), consult a physician before making dietary changes that may have negative effects. Foods used to substitute for gluten in gluten-free diets are not necessarily healthy; many are calorie-rich and nutrient-poor. Also, it's not wise to avoid all carbohydrates; some are good, and some are bad to consume. High-fiber, whole-grain carbs are very good indeed. The glycemic index (a value used to measure how much specific foods increase blood sugar levels) is not the only measure of food quality. Also consider fiber, minerals, antioxidants, and other molecules found in plants. It is better to consume the fruit than only the juice, as the juice has less fiber and may have excessive sugars. Avoid processed foods.

Good sources of fiber include the following: fruit, nuts, legumes, vegetables, brown rice, unrefined whole grains, whole wheat bread, beans, and seeds.

Animals vs. Plants

The dynamics of dietary choices are illustrated by a decision to have beefsteak with potatoes and green beans for dinner. One may feel that it is a healthy meal because of the inclusion of green beans. However, having two plant-based foods on the plate is better than just one. It's preferable if the steak is replaced with a high-fiber, vegetarian option. The steak occupies space on the plate that could have been used for something healthy. The steak is not adding anything of value to the bacteria (steak has no fiber whatsoever) and the steak is high in saturated fat.

Tofu (soybean curd) is a good source of protein and polyunsaturated fats and is cholesterol free. Tofu has essential amino acids, calcium, minerals, soy isoflavones, and other ingredients that reduce the risk of heart disease and diminish inflammation in blood vessels. Almonds, walnuts, pecans, pine nuts, hazelnuts, and peanuts are super sources of protein. Nuts and legumes also have vitamins, fiber, and minerals. Many of these dietary recommendations are helpful to decrease the risk of cancer. In short, eat a plant-based diet, low in saturated fat, with little meat.

In short, eat a plant-based diet, low in saturated fat, with little meat.

A study of 123,330 women showed that higher levels of plant protein intake was associated with lower risk of death from cardiovascular disease and stroke.[146] Whole plant foods are better than refined or processed foods. A plant-based diet is associated with a reduced risk of other chronic diseases. You probably already know this but let me say it emphatically. Eating processed foods with excess sugar and salt is a really bad idea. Such a diet has negative consequences for the gut bacteria, leading to obesity, heart disease, and diabetes.

Several scientific studies show that eating a healthy diet, rich in green leafy vegetables, berries, nuts, whole grains, and fish, will lower a person's risk of dementia. This is terrific news with zero downside. Skip the meaty sandwich and grab a salad. Skip the molasses cookie and select a nutty, granola mix. Skip the pork banh mi on doughy white bread and eat salmon for dinner.

Another reason to eat less meat: animal studies have shown it's possible to transmit systemic diseases caused by an abnormal protein configuration called amyloid through the consumption of duck liver (paté de foie gras). It is known that consumption of beef infected with bovine spongiform encephalopathy (mad cow disease) can cause an untreatable rapidly progressive dementing condition called Creutzfeldt–Jakob disease (see Chapter 7).

Mediterranean Diet

There is substantial evidence that the Mediterranean diet is a big plus to human health. The Mediterranean diet features lots of fruits, vegetables, monounsaturated fat, fish, whole grains, legumes, and nuts. It's also low in meat, dairy, saturated fat, refined grains, and alcohol consumption. My reading of the scientific literature indicates this diet may be protective against development of both Alzheimer's and Parkinson's diseases.

In addition, the Mediterranean diet has fewer precursors of the metabolite trimethylamine (TMA), leading to lower blood levels of trimethylamine oxide (TMAO), and TMAO increases vascular damage. As you may recall from earlier in the book (Chapter 9), TMA is oxidized in the liver to TMAO. Both are bad and potentially damaging. These molecules accelerate the impairment of cardiac and brain blood vessels, leading to heart attacks and possibly stroke and Alzheimer's disease.

A green Mediterranean diet may be even better than a Mediterranean diet featuring larger amounts of red and processed meat.[147] Research has shown that people who developed dementia were more likely to eat processed meats such as sausages, cured meats, and patés, as well as starchy foods such as potatoes, large amounts of alcohol, and snacks like cookies and cakes.[148] Study participants with the greatest adherence to the Mediterranean diet had the lowest risk of cognitive impairment. A high consumption of fish, vegetables, and olive oil appear to have a protective effect. The consumption of fish has been reported to decrease the risk of Alzheimer's disease associated with the apolipoprotein E (APOE) gene.

Fish

Fish is certainly preferred over beef or pork. Fatty fish have omega-3 polyunsaturated fatty acids (PUFAs) that are beneficial for health and memory. Omega-3 PUFAs are anti-inflammatory and may help relieve depression. The unsaturated fats found in fish are beneficial and fish are low in saturated fat and high in protein – they are also good sources of vitamins and minerals.

Which fish are best? Salmon, herring, lake trout, and freshwater whitefish are rich in omega-3 PUFAs. Catfish and shrimp are low in PUFAs. Smart readers can guess what I'm going to write next: minimize consumption of fish and chips, which are fried, breaded, fatty, and delicious. Minimize consumption does not mean only on Fridays. It means monthly or yearly.

There are some large fish you may want to avoid due to the risk of mercury poisoning. Those fish include swordfish, shark, mackerel, or tilefish. These fish should not be consumed regularly. Farmed fish may contain more pesticides than wild fish.

Sugar

Through billions of dollars spent on marketing by cola conglomerates, candy manufacturers, and our mothers and grandmothers who showed their love to us by baking cookies and pies, we've become addicted to sugar. Yet, please listen to me on this. It is best to limit the amount of sugar you eat and drink.

Sugar consumption is growing worldwide, leading to a big jump in the prevalence of diabetes and obesity. Excess consumption of sugar can lead to diabetes and is a risk factor for decreased cognitive function.

Excess consumption of sugar can lead to diabetes and is a risk factor for decreased cognitive function.

Some nutritional experts have suggested that sugar may be the tobacco of the current era. History professor Yuval Harari suggests that sugar is now more dangerous than gunpowder because it kills more people. Cola companies, he says, pose a far deadlier threat than al-Qaeda.[149] Diabetes and obesity shorten lives and kill. It's really that simple.

The negative effects of excess sugar consumption include the following

- inflammation and free radical production,

- obesity,
- diabetes (impaired insulin responsiveness),
- kidney and heart disease,
- gout,
- non-alcoholic fatty liver disease,
- dental cavities,
- decreased bone health, and
- leaky gut (poor integrity of the gut blood barrier).

Consumption of sugary soda has been shown to impair blood flow to the kidney and is a risk factor for cardiovascular disease and obesity. In a study of more than 100,000 women, consumption of one or more sugary drinks per day was coupled with a 42 percent greater chance of having cardiovascular disease.[150] Another study of 1,209 elders in Malaysia found that sugar intake from all sources was associated with cognitive impairment.[151] Here's still more evidence: people who drink sodas daily are 23 percent more likely to have cardiovascular disease (compared to those who rarely or never drink sugary beverages).[152] Furthermore, consumption of sodas can limit the absorption of minerals necessary for bone health.

Here's how little sugar the American Heart Association recommends you eat daily: six teaspoons a day for women and nine teaspoons a day for men. The average American far exceeds those recommendations by eating and drinking more than 20 teaspoons of sugar daily.

You might be thinking, "What if I just switch to Diet Coke or Diet Pepsi?" I wouldn't. Artificial sweeteners should also be avoided because of their effect on bacterial populations in the gut, which may change blood insulin levels and impair the control of blood glucose levels. The host microbiome may be altered by artificial sweeteners to increase the risk of diabetes and weight gain. Artificial sweeteners have also been associated with the risk of heart disease.

Televised sporting events often feature adverts for sports drinks like Gatorade. This isn't by chance. The owners of sports drinks want us to think of their product as healthy. They're often not. Sports drinks may contain excessive sugar. The electrolytes the drinks provide are not needed by most athletes. It is best to get electrolytes from food. Many sports drinks also have artificial sweeteners, colors, and flavors. Many of these unneeded additives are designated GRAS, or "generally recognized as safe," by the US Food and Drug Administration. GRAS doesn't mean that they are actually safe. Note that the designation is not ADTBS, or "actually demonstrated to be safe." Many of these additives may very well be carcinogenic or hazardous in other ways. The best approach is this: chemicals are not people; they are not entitled to be presumed innocent until proven guilty.

Evolution has provided us with a special appreciation of sweet things because sugar is a good supply of quick energy. Intake of sweet things is fine, within reason. It's helpful to consider what makes consumption of food or drink pleasing. I have asked this of lots of people and the most common response is that the quality of the food or drink is paramount (e.g., a fine wine, a spicy chicken tikka masala). This view is certainly erroneous and does not consider the functions of the nervous system. The most important determinant of the quality of an experience of eating or drinking is not the material taken in, but the context surrounding its consumption. That is, if I eat one Belgian chocolate, I will find it to be delicious. If I have already eaten ten, the eleventh may make me sick.

Years ago, I got lost on a summer hike in a desert canyon. I had little water, which I quickly drank. It took me five hours to find my way out of the canyon. As you might expect, when I reached a water fountain, I was profoundly thirsty. The taste of that water was outrageously delicious. I doubt that at that moment I would have preferred a 1976

Cote de Rhone wine; water was already magnificent. The quality of the experience of drinking was determined by my need, not only by the substance consumed.

I have emphasized this point because we can make these features of our experience of eating and drinking work for us. If reduced caloric intake is desired, skipping breakfast or lunch may improve the experience of eating the next meal. If you gradually lower your consumption of sugar your sensory faculties will change and you will develop an increased perception of the sweetness of fruit. Instead of putting sugar on your cereal in the morning, consider using raisins, which have natural sweetness and antioxidants – and fiber as well!

Snacking

It is not enough to eat healthy foods: it is critical to have a diverse assortment of healthy foods. When considering a snack, it's smart to reach for a high-fiber snack, such as raisins, dried figs, dates, or dried apricots. It is best to avoid processed foods which are often high in salt and sugar. Also, additives should be avoided such as artificial color, artificial sweeteners, preservatives, and artificial flavors. Several of these chemicals are known to cause cancer.

It is not enough to eat healthy foods: it is critical to have a diverse assortment of healthy foods.

Antioxidants

Free radicals are unstable atoms that zip around inside your body, causing damage. Antioxidants can combat free radicals. They do such a good job at hunting down free radicals that some people have dubbed antioxidants "free radical scavengers."

You can load up on antioxidants naturally by eating berries, plums, avocados, oranges, grapes, cherries, kale, spinach, and other leafy, green vegetables. Eating these foods can also reduce inflammation in the body.[153]

Antioxidants benefit us in other ways. The antioxidant content of fruits has been linked to their coloring; often, the color of fruits is caused by flavonoids that help the plant resist oxidative damage by sunlight and attract pollinators (such as the redness of strawberries or raspberries). When you eat these fruits, they protect you from the oxidative damage caused by your metabolism. The microbiota help to enable absorption of the flavonoids in the diet. Flavonoids in fruit and vegetables also have anti-amyloid as well as anti-inflammatory properties.[154] Intake of flavonoids has been reported to be protective against the development of Alzheimer's disease. Spices such as ginger, chilli, and turmeric also have anti-inflammatory properties. Saturated fatty acids have pro-inflammatory effects and omega-3 PUFAs decrease inflammatory markers. Eating fruit and vegetables can help inhibit inflammation. Fruits also have large amounts of fiber and vitamin C.

Natural Foods

When shopping, beware of the "natural" label on food. The US Food and Drug Administration does not regulate the use of the word "natural" in the marketing of food. *Natural products are not necessarily safe.* Cobra venom is completely natural but isn't safe – you wouldn't stir it into your coffee. Many things sold in health food stores are both natural and potentially dangerous. It's important that your doctor is aware of all the pills you take, including natural products and supplements. One example of a natural product that may not be good for you is coconut oil, which is high in saturated fat and has been shown to increase low-density lipoprotein cholesterol ('bad" cholesterol) and also increase cardiovascular risk. There's no firm evidence that coconut oil helps prevent Alzheimer's disease, dementia, or other diseases.[155] The American Heart Association has advised against the consumption of coconut oil.

"Everything in Moderation"?

I often hear people use the phrase, "Everything in moderation." This phrase can be quite dangerous, especially in combination with denial. For example, there's no safe level of cigarette smoking, lead poisoning, or mercury exposure. All are cumulative and can lead to brain damage and death.

It's important to define the term "moderation." You might define moderation as eating a fatty meal once a week. Or you might define moderation as eating a fatty meal once a month. Let's say that the fatty meal is a pastrami sandwich with more than 1,000 calories, 21 grams of saturated fat, and 3 grams of sodium. If you're obese, have high cholesterol, and a family history of early cardiac death, you shouldn't eat pastrami sandwiches at all.

For those without health problems, keep in mind that indulgences can get you in trouble.

Vitamins and Minerals

Vitamins are critical for the function of the brain and nervous system. The best place to get vitamins is in food.

Let's begin with B vitamins. Thiamine (B1) is an essential B vitamin and is important for the brain. It's usually only deficient in people with alcoholism, malabsorption, or other serious nutritional deficiencies. Vitamin B1 may be found in fortified cereals, fish, lentils, green peas, yogurt, and may enhance immunity, aid bone health, and reduce heart disease risk.

Pyridoxine (vitamin B6) and folic acid (vitamin B9) are also important for brain functioning. Vitamin B6 is found in fish, poultry, meat, nuts, legumes, potatoes, and whole grains. Folic acid is found in animal products, dark leafy vegetables, whole-grain cereals, and fortified grains (in the United States).

Dietary intake of vitamin A, vitamin K, magnesium, zinc, and copper have been associated with reduced heart disease. Vitamin A is present in orange and yellow fruits, carrots, dark greens, and eggs. Vitamin K is found in green leafy vegetables, collard greens, spinach, shellfish, seeds, and nuts. Zinc is found in oysters, crab, lobster, poultry, beans, and nuts. Vitamin K2 is found in fermented foods and chicken.

Vitamin B12 is very important for the central and peripheral nervous systems. It is essential for the proper functioning of nervous tissue, cannot be synthesized by humans, and is relatively difficult to absorb, because it requires a molecule to be secreted by the stomach for its absorption. Many people are deficient in vitamin B12 because of a problem in the gastrointestinal tract of which they are not aware.

Vitamin B12 may be deficient in vegetarians and is found in liver, meat, milk, poultry, fish, and eggs. Although vitamin B12 is found in multivitamin supplements, the dose is often not enough for persons who have difficulty absorbing the vitamin. Recently, high levels of dietary vitamin B12 have been associated with breast and lung cancer. It is best to have your blood level of vitamin B12 measured to see if supplementation is needed.

Blood levels of vitamin B12, B6, and folic acid are linked to a normal amino acid called homocysteine, which is present in blood.[156] Some studies show that low vitamin B12 levels are associated with Alzheimer's disease. High levels of homocysteine have been linked to heart disease, oxidative stress, stroke, and Alzheimer's disease. Fortunately, homocysteine levels can frequently be lowered by taking dietary supplements of vitamins B12, B6, and folic acid. There is evidence, which is currently incomplete, that suggests lowering homocysteine with vitamin supplementation may lower the risk of cognitive impairment in aging. It is recommended that everyone has their levels of vitamins D, B6, B12, and homocysteine monitored.

In a preliminary study, vitamin B3 has been found to be deficient in both mouse models and humans with ALS.[157] This vitamin may also inhibit cognitive loss and neurodegeneration in mouse models of Alzheimer's.[158] Vitamin B3 is found in poultry, eggs, dairy products, eggs, fish, nuts, seeds, legumes, avocados, and whole grains.

Vitamin D is important for the immune system and for calcium absorption and bone density. Studies show that over 70 percent of people in North America are deficient in vitamin D. Everyone should know their serum vitamin D level because of its importance in bone health and the immune system. As discussed in Chapter 5, the immune system is highly involved in brain disorders in aging, as well as heart disease and stroke. Magnesium may be helpful in absorption of vitamin D. Vitamin D is synthesized in the body when exposed to sunlight, but it's also available in fatty fish, liver, beef, egg yolks, and mushrooms.

Vitamin E has a potent ability to counteract free radicals[159] and is found in brown rice, nuts, seeds, vegetable oils, green leafy vegetables, and fortified cereals. Recently, it was reported that vitamin E and C intake may be protective against Parkinson's disease.

For most people, multivitamins are not proven to improve health.[160] Actually, people who use multivitamins are often already those with a healthy diet. Multivitamins can help people with dietary deficiencies, alcoholism, or poor absorption of nutrients. Supplements can be harmful, at times – beta-carotene supplements have been reported to increase the risk of lung cancer in smokers. Taking vitamin E and antioxidant supplements may increase the risk of some cancers. However, it is good to consume them in food.

Minerals are important for metabolism and the health of bones, heart, muscles, and the brain. Minerals include calcium, phosphorus, sodium, potassium, magnesium, manganese, sulfur, chloride, iron, iodine, fluoride, zinc, copper, selenium, chromium, and cobalt. They may be found in nuts, seeds, shellfish, vegetables, eggs, beans, avocados, berries, and yogurt. Minerals are also found in organ meats, but it is not necessary to eat meat to have adequate minerals in your diet.

Magnesium deficiency is common and may impair immune function. Magnesium is found in deep ocean fish, seeds, nuts, whole-grain foods, dark-green vegetables, fruits, and dark chocolate. Supplements of magnesium may be toxic in high doses. Calcium intake is important for bone and muscle health, blood clotting, and the avoidance of osteoporosis.

Polyphenols and Bioflavonoids

Polyphenols are a class of molecules that contain multiple phenol groups. Joseph Lister (1827–1912) demonstrated the power of a compound called carbolic acid in the late-nineteenth century. Carbolic acid, also known as phenol, was the first effective and widely used antiseptic agent. It allowed the field of surgery to greatly lower mortality rates. The story of Lister and carbolic acid is well told in Lindsey Fitzharris' *The Butchering Art: Joseph Lister's Quest to Transform the Grisly World of Victorian Medicine*. Carbolic acid has one phenol group and is biologically powerful.

Bioflavonoids are polyphenols found in plants, and they have many powerful effects on microbes (and humans too). Flavonoids have many desirable health effects, including anti-amyloid actions and lowering of blood pressure. They may also inhibit clumping and spreading of disease-related brain proteins. Flavonoids are found in fruit, vegetables, cereals, tea and coffee, spices, berries, beans, nuts, soy as well as red wine.

Flavonoids help give color to plants, protecting them from the Sun and attracting pollinators such as insects, flies, and birds. When we eat these polyphenol compounds, we take advantage of their antioxidant effects.

Curcumin, a natural polyphenol and bioflavinoid from the Asian spice turmeric, may lower inflammation.[161] It may improve the innate immune system's ability to increase clearance from the brain of toxic proteins involved in the neurodegenerative disorders.[162,163] Turmeric is very flavorful and adds lovely coloring to your meals.

Another source of polyphenols is green tea. Green tea is made from the same plant as black and oolong tea, but it is produced without the withering and oxidation process used to make those other teas. Green tea contains polyphenols, which are anti-inflammatory and reduce oxidative toxicity and blood pressure. Green tea consumption may lower low-density lipoprotein cholesterol levels, decrease periodontal disease, and cause weight loss. It has been proposed that the polyphenols in green tea may beneficially alter gut bacteria and their metabolites (the molecules that are made by the bacteria). One Japanese study found that drinking green tea may lower the risk of Alzheimer's disease.[164] Green tea has about 30 percent of the caffeine content of coffee and is safe to drink. However, avoid high doses of green tea or green-tea extract because of possible liver toxicity. Certainly two glasses of green tea a day is fine but taking green tea extract as a supplement is not recommended.

Finally, phytoestrogens are plant-derived estrogens (phyto means plant), found in soybeans, pomegranates, spinach, and other plants, which lower lipids, change the packaging of DNA, and have beneficial effects on blood clotting, blood vessel disease, and reduce the risk of Alzheimer's disease.[161,165]

Salt

Fast food is really bad for you. And one of the reasons it's bad for you is the salt. A quarter pounder with cheese from the Golden Arches has 1,140 milligrams of sodium. And most people get it with fries, which, by the way, are another 350 milligrams – taking the whole meal up to 1,490 milligrams of sodium.

The American Heart Association recommends consuming just 2,300 milligrams of sodium daily and believes most people should be eating and drinking closer to 1,500 milligrams of sodium (so that one meal from the Arches breaks that count), but most people in the United States eat and drink more than 3,400 milligrams of sodium. Be aware of your salt intake and eat less salty food.

High levels of salt intake are known to worsen hypertension. Recently, it has been learned that salt also influences the microbiota, affecting the immune system: higher levels of salt consumption accelerate inflammation in the brain and in blood vessels. A high-salt diet also diminishes the ability of white blood cells to kill bacteria and decreases the production of beneficial short-chain fatty acid production by the microbiota.

Fasting

Another dietary approach to health is intermittent fasting. This should only be done with the assistance of a physician and may not be good for people with diabetes or kidney or liver problems.

Our hunter–gatherer ancestors were not able to eat three meals a day because of the variable availability of food (they did not have stores, refrigerators, or pantries). Research has shown that periods of not eating, either during the day or on alternate days, have beneficial effects on metabolism and disease. Intermittent fasting may improve liver function and increase the production of beneficial short-chain fatty acids such as butyrate (these small molecules are made by gut bacteria and have healthful effects). The diversity of gut bacteria may also be enhanced with fasting. Fasting lowers stores of fat in the body, improves blood lipids, lowers blood pressure, improves DNA repair, and may have beneficial effects on cancer, mental health, and the regulation of blood sugar. There may also be good effects of fasting on body weight, inflammation, neurodegeneration, heart disease, and stroke.[166] Also, fasting increases the production of ketones in the blood, which may be neuroprotective, increase sensitivity to insulin, and improve cognition. Furthermore, fasting may increase brain-derived neurotrophic factor and improve resistance to stress and maintenance of functional balance (homeostasis).

The easiest approach to fasting is called intermittent fasting, in which there is a period of about 16 hours a day where there is no caloric intake. This can be from 8 p.m. at night till noon the next day. Fasting may be a problem for diabetics or those with eating disorders and it's important that fasting does not lead to feasting.

Water Balance

Hydration is an important and often ignored aspect of health. At the National Institutes of Health, my colleagues and I found that older people don't drink as much as they need – this is called "a diminished response to water deprivation." The people participating in our study spent the night at a research hospital. We told them not to drink from 9 p.m. to 8 a.m. At 8 a.m., they were given access to ice water and the amount they drank was recorded.

We found that older people in the study drank less water than they should have, as determined by blood tests. This problem was relatively more marked in persons with Alzheimer's disease.

Hydration is an important and often ignored aspect of health.

Dehydration caused by poor water intake can worsen heart and cerebrovascular disease and constipation, as well as cause cognitive impairment. Older persons should be aware of the fact that thirst may not be a reliable indicator of how much water their bodies need; they may need to drink more that than their thirst indicates.

The amount of water needed varies by individual. Discuss the situation with your doctor, as it will depend upon your health status in regard to kidney function, diabetes, and heart disease. Hydration requirements also vary based on your physical environment, physical activity level, and underlying health conditions.

How to Change Dietary Habits

It is not easy to change the way we eat. I suggest using small changes which are more likely to endure. Consider replacing juice with fruit, replacing white rice with brown rice at least once a week (or mix brown and white rice together), replacing sugar with raisins on cereal, replacing a chocolate bar with a fig and almond for a snack, replacing a hamburger with a veggie burger, and replacing a pepperoni pizza from a fast-food chain with a pizza made at home using whole wheat bread and fresh vegetables.

I suggest using small changes which are more likely to endure.

Summary of Dietary Recommendations

The lists below provide a summary of my dietary recommendations. I suggest we avoid the following:

- red meat (beef and pork),
- refined grains (white rice, white bread),
- high salt,
- poor dietary diversity,
- low-fiber content,
- processed foods,
- high saturated fat,
- excess alcohol (see Chapter 25),
- excess sugar (natural or artificial sweeteners),
- artificial colors, flavors, preservatives,
- sodas,
- fast food, and
- processed food.

Instead, make sure you have enough of the following:

- whole grains (brown rice, whole wheat bread),
- fish,
- chicken (better than beef or pork),
- high dietary diversity,
- high-fiber content (beans, whole grains, fruit, berries, vegetables, legumes, nuts),
- plant-based food,
- unprocessed food,
- tofu,
- low saturated fat,
- green leafy vegetables, and
- spices.

I hope that the concept of the opportunity of aging will assist in understanding how our food choices impact the quality of our lives as we get older. You can do it!

21 MICROBIAL CONSIDERATIONS

A reader who has little knowledge of such matters may be surprised by my recommendation to absorb large quantities of microbes, as the general belief is that microbes are all harmful. This belief, however, is erroneous. There are many useful microbes, amongst which the lactic bacilli have an honorable place. Moreover, the attempt has already been made to cure certain diseases by the administration of cultures of bacteria.

Elie Metchnikoff (1845–1916), Russian scientist

The first suggestion that intestinal bacteria may be involved in health comes from the observations of Elie Metchnikoff, an important Russian scientist and colleague of Louis Pasteur. He found that inhabitants of Bulgaria in the Caucasus mountains had a long life, which he believed was attributable to yogurt consumption. His research identified the first class of probiotic bacteria, lactobacillus, as a responsible agent. Metchnikoff won the Nobel Prize in Physiology or Medicine in 1908 (shared with German scientist Paul Ehrlich "in recognition of their work on immunity").

Metchnikoff is credited with coining the term *gerontology* (the study of aging). Ahead of his time, he once said, "Inflammation as understood in man and the higher animals is a phenomenon that almost always results from the intervention of some pathogenic microbe."[167] He would have certainly appreciated the concept emphasized in this book that microbes are involved in health as well as disease.

Microbial exposure in early life is necessary for the development of a healthy immune system.

Microbial exposure in early life is necessary for the development of a healthy immune system. Excessive cleanliness has been linked to an increasing risk of asthma and allergic condition in childhood. Microbiota researchers Jack Gilbert and Rob Knight have written a book about the importance of microbial exposure on child development, *Dirt Is Good: The Advantage of Germs for Your Child's Developing Immune System.*[120]

It is difficult to make specific recommendations concerning microbial exposures at this time. Considerable research is being done worldwide about which bacterial populations will be best to consume as probiotics (live bacteria are believed to aid health and enhance bacterial populations in the gut). However, I can recommend the steps below.

- Children should be able to play in natural environments without excessive attention to cleanliness. There is research to suggest that the immune system of children who grow up with a dog is better than that of those who do not have such exposure.
- Probiotics may be helpful, but it is not clear which are best. (Probiotics have been found to help control constipation in people with Parkinson's disease.)
- Consumption of yogurt which has live bacteria is desirable.
- Don't eat yogurt with a lot of sugar, as is often found in many yogurts. Rather than eating a yogurt with added fruit and sugar, it's better to eat plain yogurt and add your own fruit.

- Other foods that contain live bacteria that may be beneficial including kimchi (high-salt Korean fermented cabbage and radishes) and natto (Japanese fermented soybeans). Both kimchi and natto are excellent sources of vitamins and minerals.
- Prebiotics are non-digestible fibers that cannot be digested by people; they are designed for their ability to be metabolized by desirable gut bacteria. It is also not clear which prebiotics are best. Psyllium husk (also known as isabgol) is a dietary fiber which can relive constipation and enhance fiber intake. It can cause bloating if not taken with an adequate amount of water. Consumption of high-fiber foods will have a similar effect on the microbiome as prebiotics.
- Kombucha, a fermented sweetened tea drink, has probiotics and antioxidants but may be high in calories and may cause bloating. It's not clear that the bacteria in kombucha are beneficial.

22 DENTAL CARE

The mouth is home to more than 1,000 different species of microbes. These microbes live in the nose, mouth, and throat and help to protect us against invasive, disease-causing organisms. We don't have a choice about their residency in our bodies. If we wanted to remove them once and for all we would need a blow torch. That is to say, they can't be removed. Because of their contribution to disease, we must monitor and control their populations as best we can. To put it another way: we need them, and they need us.

We must be sure that they are not having a party in our mouth. The best way to avoid having an unhealthy population of organisms is to practice good oral hygiene: brush upon wakening, after meals, and at bedtime, use dental floss, and visit a dentist two or three times a year for check-ups and cleaning.

We need to take care of our oral health because it is good for our brain and heart.

We need to take care of our oral health because it is good for our brain and heart. Of course, it's also good for our teeth, but consideration of the role of oral health in brain and heart disease will help us to understand its importance to our health and fitness.

23 DEALING WITH DOCTORS AND DRUGS

One of the first duties of the physician is to educate the masses not to take medicine.

William Osler (1849–1919), author of the most important medicine textbook of the first half of the twentieth century

In order to maintain the highest level of your four reserve factors it is necessary to know how to interact with the medical professionals and the medications they prescribe. It is similarly valuable to understand and appreciate the perspective of clinical research.

The Importance of Being Heard

Some years ago, I was walking and noticed a pain in my left ankle. It worsened over several weeks and prevented me from playing tennis. I went to see a prominent orthopedist who specialized in legs and feet, at the university hospital where I work. The attendant put me in a room. I waited an hour for the doctor to arrive. He greeted me and had already been told by the nurse that I was there for pain in my left ankle. Before I could say much, he squeezed the ankle and said I should have an MRI scan. As he was leaving the room, after just a three-minute visit, I was surprised how angry I became. The doctor had shown no interest in the story of my ankle pain. As he was halfway out the door, I sternly requested he come back so I could tell him about my ankle. He did not know, nor did he appreciate the fact, that we are all entitled to our stories. To the orthopedist, I was one more ankle out of thousands. But to me, it was an important factor in my ability to walk.

Another time I was considering having a major surgery and needed to choose between five different treatment options and several potential surgeons. I chose a surgeon who looked at me, did not keep his gaze fixed on his computer, and spoke to me as a human being. Another possible surgeon did not look at me and gave me a good view only of his left ear, because he was focused on his computer. I was surprised at how angry I was that he would not address me like a human being.

These two anecdotes illustrate an important issue in dealing with medical professionals. As patients, we have the right to have our story and voice respected. Each and every one of us should be treated like human beings. Our stories are an important part of who we are. We are not machines in need of mechanical intervention. Many people are exceptionally passive in their pursuit of medical care and will accept whatever negligence, avoidance, or abuse they receive. It's up to us to be powerful advocates for our own welfare and insist on having medical professionals listen to our stories and attend to our needs. We need to be active partners in our healthcare. In order to do that we need to be assertive and speak out when necessary.

We need to be active partners in our healthcare. In order to do that we need to be assertive and speak out when necessary.

Important issues in interactions with doctors are noted below.

Choosing a Physician

Choosing the right doctor is tough. The following points are worth considering when you are faced with making a choice.

- Naturally, we are attracted to doctors who are friendly, thoughtful, and kind. But a doctor with good bedside manners might not be the doctor you need. It's possible that the doctor with poor bedside manner may be the best choice. An important determinant here is how acute or important is the issue you're facing.
- Physicians involved in teaching are generally better informed than those who are not, since the demands of teaching require physicians to stay up to date. Physicians who teach are more likely to have time to attend to their own education. Also, physicians who publish are often better educated than those who don't. I admit that I am seriously biased in regard to this preference for academic physicians. Certainly, there are many outstanding physicians who are not teachers and do not publish.
- The doctor at an academic medical center is subject to higher standards than most physicians. At a university, physicians must participate in patient care, teaching, research, and publishing to get promoted. Academic physicians are often paid by salary, not by the number of patients they treat. Many doctors in community settings are paid by the amount of clinical work they accomplish or the number of referrals produced (e.g., if they take a week off to go to a conference, they will have no income for that week).
- If possible, find out what people who work with physicians say about them, including other doctors, nurses, medical assistants, technicians, administrative assistants, and administrators.
- Just because a doctor works in another city doesn't mean they're better than one around the corner. Beware of the belief that someone local could not possibly be good, and that someone far away must be excellent because of where they work. This is often not an effective strategy.

- Make appointments only with board-certified physicians. Board certification is a minimum qualification – it does not require excellence, only a minimum level of competence. There is no excuse for a practicing physician to not be board certified. (Being board eligible implies that the physician is qualified to take the board exam but has not yet taken it or hasn't passed the exam yet.)
- Remember, about 50 percent of physicians are below average. If a medical school graduates 150 doctors, whoever occupies the position of bottom of the class will certainly find a job! Of course, no one will have access to this information, but this is a solid warning that we all need to be active partners in the pursuit of our health and fitness.
- If possible, be aware of conflicts of interest. A surgeon may be evaluated by their practice in regard to financial productivity. How many operations are they doing? A cardiologist might earn more money by recommending more surgeries. If a physician doesn't recommend enough surgeries (and other procedures), they may not be rehired or promoted. This problem is reviewed in the book *Heart Health*.[168]
- As a patient, ask questions at every visit. Don't let the doctor sneak out of the room when you're not looking, followed by the nurse saying, "You can go now."
- Interpret online reviews with skepticism. Doctors with good bedside manners may have good reviews, even though they are incompetent.
- Beware of specialists, subspecialists, and super-sub-specialists. Have you heard about the specialist who said during their career that they learned more and more about less and less, until they knew absolutely everything about nothing? This is related to how acute and important the problem is. If you have a sore throat, you don't need an otolaryngologist (ear, nose,

and throat specialist). If you have a rare disease, the best person for you to see may be at the National Institutes of Health in Bethesda Maryland, at the National Hospital for Neurology and Neurosurgery in London, England, or at another top academic medical center. However, although specialists can often provide the critical care you need, their narrow vision may impair their understanding of the whole situation.

People are complex creatures. And disease is complex. Reading about your condition may help, but you must understand that to write about disease, the writer must simplify. And the information may be misleading or erroneous.

To treat disease, a doctor must understand complex, interrelated specifics. Science is advancing with great speed. For example, by spring of 2021, the National Library of Medicine featured 119,201 papers dedicated to coronavirus disease 2019 (Covid-19), a virus not known to exist less than two years earlier. It is also the case that some things written in textbooks are wrong by the time the textbook is published. Reading up for yourself is not enough. These are good reasons to obtain expert guidance when consulting a physician concerning serious disease.

Discussing Your Medication with Your Physician

When it comes to discussing medications with your physician, the following suggestions may be helpful to consider.

- Bring all your medications, supplements, and vitamins with you to every visit with a physician. Make sure the physician is aware of everything you take (medications, supplements, vitamins, herbal preparations, ethnic remedies, gastrointestinal aids). They should review this list comprehensively at each visit (see Case Study 10).

- If medications are prescribed, make certain you understand their indications, side effects, dosing schedule, possible interactions with other drugs, and whether the drug needs to be taken on an empty stomach or with food.
- If a physician suggests that you take a new drug, read about the drug at home and understand its effects, as far as possible.
- Jot down your questions in advance and bring paper and pencil with you so you can make notes while discussing your condition.
- If an illness or disease threatens disability or death, consider getting second or third opinions, including a referral to academic medical centers.
- If you don't understand what the doctor is saying, ask for explanations. The visit may be stressful and you may be tempted to avoid that by leaving at the earliest opportunity. Still, it's best to take advantage of the chance to find out what you need to know and what you need to do.
- Be aware of the powerful factor of denial of illness. No one wants to be sick; this is human nature. It's better to confront a problem directly than to ignore it.
- Make sure the physician gives you their opinion before you leave. This opinion must include what the physician thinks is going on and what they think should be done. These opinions should make sense. For example, if you bring in a 76-year-old parent with a memory problem and the doctor says they thinks the diagnosis is "senile dementia," you know you need another doctor. As I've said, the phrase "senile dementia" is obsolete – it is also not a diagnosis. It merely indicates that the person is old (you know that already) and the person has the symptoms and signs suggestive of dementia (you may already know that as well). But what is necessary is to know the cause of the problem.

- Family history is an important part of the medical encounter. Be prepared to discuss the health histories of your parents, siblings, children, aunts, uncles, and grandparents.

Case Study 10

A 74-year-old hypertensive diabetic man was seen by me for paranoid behavior and loss of memory for one year. He thought that people were hiding things and "trying to put things over on him." He also complained of an altered sense of smell and taste. Two years earlier, he had a colostomy for cancer of the colon. His only medication was an oral antidiabetic agent. An examination showed that he had poor abstraction, judgment, word finding, and decision making. Routine blood tests were normal. MRI of the brain showed one small stroke. He worked as a manager of a ball bearing factory. Because of the possibility of toxic exposure at work, a panel of tests for heavy-metal poisoning was completed. It revealed he had a toxic level of the metal bismuth in his blood. Bismuth is known to be an uncommon cause of cognitive impairment. It was subsequently learned that he used a product called bismuth subgallate as a colostomy deodorant. He had not informed anyone about it, because it was not a drug. The product was a deodorant, and we had asked him specifically what drugs he was taking. Because of the discovery of this toxic exposure, he stopped using the bismuth product and he was markedly improved six months later. He had no further paranoid behavior, complaints of memory loss, or difficulty with executive functioning. His ability to smell and taste returned. To enhance awareness of the potential toxicity for this therapy we published this case in the journal *Clinical Neuropharmacology*.[169]

> It's critical that healthcare providers are aware of all items being taken, including medications, supplements, vitamins, herbal agents, folk remedies, and other products.

Physicians and Medical Errors

Physicians sometimes make mistakes. Any activity involving human behavior will have errors. In 1999, NASA sent a space vehicle to Mars with the parachute switches installed upside down. Undoubtedly, NASA has the smartest space engineers anywhere, but they made a serious error. On at least two occasions, an American neurosurgeon has operated on the wrong side of someone's head (the doctor was looking at the MRI scan of the wrong person). In 2021, an 82-year-old Austrian man had his right leg amputated above the knee when the procedure he needed was a left leg amputation. The mistake was attributed to human error.

The lesson here is that regardless of the eminence of the physician you visit, or researcher whose paper you read, it is possible that person is wrong. Thus, it is critical to remain involved, observant, and ask questions. And then ask more questions! In summary, *you should be an active participant in your own care and fierce in the pursuit of what's best for you* (see Case Study 11).

The Importance of Considering the Whole Person

Be aware of the need for coordination. Many people have several subspecialists dealing with various parts of the body, but nobody to be aware of the interactions among these body parts and among the subspecialists. Everyone needs one physician to be responsible for the whole person.

This individual should also be responsible for dealing with all the subspecialists and seeing that the whole person is not lost in the melee. Our interdependent parts cannot be considered without awareness of the whole person!

Case Study 11

Many years ago, I got a call from my mother's 86-year-old cousin, Elsie. She had had a headache and loss of vision in her right eye, which had come on suddenly a few days before. I was immediately concerned this could be a kind of vascular inflammation in blood vessels serving the eye in older persons, which can cause severe visual impairment and potentially blindness (called temporal arteritis). I called her physician and explained that I was a neurology resident and wanted to know if he had tested her for temporal arteritis and prescribed steroids to diminish the risk of her other eye being involved. He told me that she was already blind in her right eye and that giving her steroids would not help because it was too late. I called the most experienced neurologist I knew and got her an appointment to see him the next day. Then I called Elsie and said she needed to be treated for a serious vascular problem that could affect the vision in her other eye as well and that I had gotten her an appointment the next day with an accomplished physician. She told me that she trusted her doctor, that he had been taking care of her for over 40 years and she could not possibly go see anyone else. I told her there was a serious risk she would go blind if she did not follow my advice. I also said her doctor was seriously mistaken and did not know what he was doing. She did not go to see the neurologist I had found for her and did not get placed on the steroids she needed. Two weeks later, she lost her vision in the other eye. Within one year she had fallen, broken her hip, and died.

We must realize our opinion of physicians often is based on their joviality, conviviality, verbal skills, and salesmanship. All of these qualities are remote from the skills of being well informed and having good decision-making abilities.

Medication Interactions

Medications can cure disease, but they can also cause it. Prescription drugs are the commonest cause of reversible mental impairment. Negative effects of drugs on the brain can be caused by the drug itself, as well as interactions with other drugs, food intake, kidney dysfunction, smoking, alcohol, poor hydration, drug expiration, and the microbiota. A drug may work well when taken alone but may no longer be effective when a second drug is added because it interferes with the absorption and metabolism of the first drug. About one-quarter of non-antibiotic drugs influence gut bacteria.

Medications can cure disease, but they can also cause it.

Older people are often taking several medications that may interact to have negative effects on the brain and cause cognitive impairment. Polypharmacy is the concurrent use of five or more medications for one or many conditions.[170] The occurrence of polypharmacy is increasing around the world, and more than half of older people may be exposed.[171] This is an especially important problem in older people who may have many conditions requiring treatment. The risk of cognitive impairment is higher in people taking more than five medications, compared to those taking fewer than five.[170] Nearly 50 percent of older people are taking one or more drugs that aren't medically needed.[171]

Many physicians are not aware of the special needs of older people. In particular, it is known that physicians commonly prescribe drugs which impair memory functions in healthy older persons. The number of neurons in the brain that use the neurotransmitter acetylcholine is reduced in aging; these neurons, referred to as cholinergic, are critical for memory and learning. As a result, many older people can develop cognitive losses as a consequence of taking drugs that interfere with the function of acetylcholine in the brain, even though younger people can safely take the drugs.[172]

The use of anticholinergic agents as well as benzodiazepine drugs can increase the risk of dementia. Benzodiazepines, which include psychoactive drugs such as diazepam and alprazolam, pose a special risk for the production of cognitive impairment in older persons. Benzodiazepines produce dependence and impair memory, attention, and motor abilities. They also increase accident rates and mortality. Some benzodiazepines have a slow half-life and toxic blood levels can easily be reached when they are taken every day (see Case Study 4).

The risk that a person is not taking their medication properly is about 30 percent when they are taking one drug. If they take ten drugs, the odds are well over 90 percent that they are not taking them properly (poor compliance). This is an enormous cause of illness, disability, and death worldwide.

It's extremely important for people to discuss drugs and the potential for drug interactions with their doctor. When taking medications, it's also important to do it as prescribed. If a drug is designed to be taken with food, it is more likely to have side effects and not be effective if it is taken on an empty stomach. People need to educate themselves about the drugs they're taking and ask questions when uncertain.

People need to educate themselves about the drugs they're taking and ask questions when uncertain.

The significance of interactions of bodily systems in aging is well illustrated regarding drugs. Older people experience reductions in all these areas: muscle mass, blood volume, plasma proteins, liver function, cholinergic neurons, cerebral blood flow, lung capacity, cerebral metabolism, diversity of gut bacteria, and kidney function. At the same time, they also have alterations in drug distribution and metabolism. Gut bacteria play important roles in metabolizing drugs, as well as influencing their absorption. In addition, alcohol intake can also influence drug absorption as well as metabolism.

Older people have a heightened baseline risk of altered heart rhythm from medications, as well as central nervous system complications and drug interactions. The binding of drugs in the blood may also be impaired, as well as the reduced breakdown of the drug by the liver, kidney, and the microbiota. And at the same time, older people are often taking many drugs that interact with each other for absorption, metabolism, and mechanism of action.

It is particularly critical for all medications to be reviewed regularly. Many people are taking many drugs they no longer need. It is a responsibility of the physician at each visit to review all medications. Unfortunately, physicians may not look at the medication list. Or the physician may feel that they can't review drugs prescribed by a specialist in a different discipline.

Many people are taking many drugs they no longer need.

It is important to recognize that many drugs cannot be discontinued suddenly but must rather be tapered slowly. It is necessary to pay attention to expiration dates of drugs because, with time, they may become inactive and, on occasion, develop new toxic features.

The evaluation of new drugs can be difficult. Drug companies have a complex and conflicted relationship with the regulatory agencies and their committees. There are also frequently conflicts amongst drug study investigators, drug companies, and medical journals. Because of these complexities, it can be difficult for physicians to evaluate the safety, efficacy, and cost-effectiveness of new drugs. It is best for people to read about the medications they're taking and talk to their doctor and, if necessary, the drug companies, to have their questions addressed. If your doctor is not happy with you asking detailed questions about drugs you've have been prescribed, find another doctor.

Cost is certainly an important consideration. In general, generic drugs cost less and are equally safe and effective as those still under patent protection. It is not uncommon for a new drug to be considerably more expensive than a generic version or a different lower-cost drug, even though the new drug is not significantly better. It's good to be cautious about new drugs promising to alleviate many problems. As they say, the devil is in the details. Too often, drug companies make it difficult to understand the details involved.

In considering the use of new drugs, it is worthwhile to be aware of another source of bias. Because of the need to be relieved of disease, and the suffering experienced, we may all have our judgment clouded by bias toward favorable expectations. This bias is difficult to remove but can best be dealt with through an awareness that our judgment may be influenced by this prejudice.

Many drugs and supplements are sold because of false claims of beneficial effects on memory. So-called nootropic agents, which claim to enhance cognition, attention, and memory, have been tested and do not work. Ginkgo has been tested for Alzheimer's disease and found not to enhance performance. Fish oil supplements have also been found to have no significant effect on cognition. Prevagen is another agent sold as a dietary-supplement memory aid, which has not been demonstrated to be effective in clinical trials. Many similar substances are likely not to enter the brain well or be absorbed in the stomach. The purported "active ingredient" of Prevagen is apoaequorin, which is extracted from jellyfish. It is not known if the compound enters the brain. Prevagen has been advertised heavily as originating from jellyfish, as if we all know the long list of effective jellyfish-related products (I am not aware of them). It claims to be the No. 1 pharmacist-recommended agent for memory enhancement. I made several calls to the manufacturer of Prevagen and was not able to speak with someone to answer my questions: What is the half-life of apoaequorin in the blood? Does it enter the brain? How many pharmacists were involved in reporting their No. 1 ranking?

In a 2020 legal settlement, Quincy Bioscience, the maker of Prevagen, agreed "to resolve the claims that it misrepresented its Prevagen products as supporting brain health and helping with memory loss."

Vaccines

It is important to be properly vaccinated against infectious diseases. Many vaccines need to be regularly updated. The risk of infectious disease is considerably higher in older compared to younger persons. Vaccinations are an excellent way to enhance our physical reserve factor through immunological mechanisms.

Covid-19 has a significantly higher rate of serious illness and death in older persons. The Covid-19 vaccines that are now administered worldwide are highly effective and safe. Herpes zoster (also known as shingles) is a debilitating and painful condition that may be chronic. The opportunity to prevent or diminish its severity should not be lost. Therefore, everyone over the age of 50 or 60 should have the new herpes zoster vaccine (Shingrix), which significantly diminishes the occurrence and severity of herpes zoster infections. (Persons who are immunosuppressed, have HIV/AIDS, are receiving radiation, chemotherapy, or have hematological illnesses may not be suitable for the herpes zoster vaccination.)

Infectious conditions which can be avoided with the help of vaccines include the following: Covid-19; hepatitis A and B; herpes zoster (shingles); influenza (seasonal flu); measles; meningococcal meningitis; mumps; pneumococcal pneumonia; and tetanus, diphtheria, and pertussis (vaccines usually administered together).

Understanding Research

In the words of Louis Pasteur, the French chemist and discoverer of the germ theory of disease:[173]

> *Preconceived ideas are like searchlights which illumine the path of the experimenter and serve him as a guide to interrogate nature. They become a danger only if he transforms them into fixed ideas. This is why I should like to see these profound words inscribed on the threshold of all the temples of science: "The greatest derangement of the mind is to believe in something because one wishes it to be so."*

We live in a remarkable time where information is free and immediately available. But much of this information is wrong. This includes tweets, Facebook postings, YouTube videos, as well as articles published in peer-reviewed scientific literature. This is an especially important problem in the area of Alzheimer's disease because it is a subject of great public interest. Thus, journalists are eager to run stories about new approaches to the disease. Many reporters elevate the importance of new studies even when those studies have not been well documented or repeated. Scientists are at fault too. Some researchers feel the pressure to publish before others. This leads to the publication of premature and incomplete results that often cannot be replicated, which is key to showing that an alleged finding is true.

What is important is to have a high degree of suspicion and evaluate evidence, not anecdotes.

There are no simple answers to this problem. Certainly, articles published in peer-reviewed scientific journals are more reliable than those reported in newspapers, magazines, and shared on social media. What is important is to have a high degree of suspicion and evaluate evidence, not anecdotes. Assessing evidence is made more difficult by the understandable need to find solutions. Appreciating the presence of this form of bias is necessary, so that reasonable judgments can be made. In evaluating press reports, find out where the work was done and what is the evidence. If the new approach is said to be applicable to all human conditions (aches and pains, impotence, hair growth, etc.), it probably isn't valid. If there are no side effects and it's 100 percent safe, it's likely 100 percent ineffective.

Research Registries and Trials

Participation in research registries or trials can be of great value to patients. The best example is the drug zidovudine, the first effective antiretroviral medication for the treatment of HIV/AIDS. The drug was first described in 1964 but was not approved by the US Food and Drug Administration until 1987. Before its approval, the only people able to receive this effective agent were those in clinical trials. By participating in clinical trials, patients may have an opportunity to receive an effective medication several years before it is available to the public.

Clinical trials evaluating the effect of drugs that are designed to improve performance or modify disease progression in Alzheimer's disease have been under way for several decades. Unfortunately, nearly all trials in the past decade or so have not helped bring forth an effective remedy. Several trials have focused on removing amyloid plaques in the brain through immunological mechanisms. These studies have been successful in modifying the target molecules. However, there has not been significant improvement in the lives of people. In some cases, patients with Alzheimer's disease participating in studies have suffered significant complications in research trials.

Hopefully, new studies will identify agents that are able to modify the onset and progression of neurodegenerative diseases. A wide array of new approaches to Alzheimer's disease treatment is now being pursued. There is considerable work under way on the use of drugs, antibiotics, antibodies, vaccines, prebiotics, probiotics, and medical foods that can alter the microbiome to impair disease mechanisms.

It is important to consider that participants in research registries may have an opportunity to receive truly effective agents before government approval. When an effective drug is developed, the first people to get it will be those participating in a clinical trial. Others may need to wait three or four years before it is approved and becomes widely available (assuming of course that the agent is found to be effective). It may be many years before such a truly effective drug is discovered, but it is impossible to know when this will happen. Participation in research registries in clinical trials is completely voluntary and should be at no cost. Subjects can resign from a trial at any time. It's important to remember that participants in clinical trials are taking an unproven drug that may not help.

Research on age-related diseases such as Alzheimer's disease has largely depended on experiments involving laboratory animals. Many interventions that work well on lab mice don't work on humans. Several treatments involving cooling and medications have successfully minimized the effect of head and spinal cord injury in mice, but not in humans. Notably, mice live only one to two years, so we shouldn't be surprised if a disease in mice doesn't completely mimic human conditions. We must appreciate that studies of human aging take a long time.

There's also an overwhelming bias in science to create experiments using simpler models. The interest in smaller and smaller organisms and cells and molecules has gotten a bit out of control. It can be difficult for researchers studying human subjects to compete for grants and publications with scientists studying animal models.

The value of animal models must be recognized but the focus must remain on human problems. After all, most US scientists studying aging-related disorders obtain funding from the National Institutes of Health, and not from the NIMB (the National Institute of Mouse Biology). (No, such an institute does not actually exist.)

A key word, once more, is diversity. Difficult scientific problems require diverse approaches. Frequently, molecular mechanisms can be studied in animal or cellular models that cannot be investigated in human subjects now.

Artificial intelligence is advancing very quickly to develop the ability to use computer modeling to complete investigations that would have required animal studies in the past. Great progress has recently been made with computer modeling in understanding the way proteins fold into complex structures. This work will undoubtedly have a great impact on the development of drugs to treat age-related disorders.

Research in animals requires consideration of the assumptions that are made. After all, mice are not little men in white fur suits. However, about 85 percent of the genes in mice are similar to those in humans and the basic biochemistry concerning glucose metabolism and neurotransmitters are similar. Fruit flies (*Drosophila melanogaster*) are exceptionally simple organisms but their biological processes model those of humans very precisely. Six Nobel Prizes have been awarded for research on these animals. Seventy-five percent of the genes responsible for human diseases have similar genes in flies. In 2021, I worked on fruit fly models of amyotrophic lateral sclerosis (ALS) with colleagues in Kyoto, Japan. We studied the effects of exposure to bacterial products on the signs of the disease in the flies. This research is under way at the time of this writing.

George E. P. Box, a British statistician, is quoted as saying "All models are wrong, but some are useful." This seems to me to be very apt.

24 HAZARDOUS BEHAVIORS

It is important to avoid injuries at all stages of life. Older people are at a relatively higher risk of developing injuries as well as dying from injuries, compared to younger people. Falling is an important cause of death amongst older persons. The risk of hip fracture increases exponentially with age in both men and women. It is reported that 30% of people with a hip fracture will die in the following year.[174] Dietary measures to reduce the risk of osteoporosis may help. Physical exercise can also build stronger bones and muscles.

Driving is important for functional independence and development and the maintenance of social relationships. However, older people with or without dementia may develop impaired driving performance. Research from our group at the National Institutes of Health and others has shown that many older persons and those with cognitive impairment often do not stop driving until they have had a crash. Cognitively impaired persons may have particular trouble with turns against traffic, because that task involves an assessment of the speed of oncoming traffic. It is a good sign that a person should stop driving if a family member is afraid to be in the car with the older driver. It is wise to drive with the person to assess their function and also to discuss the matter with a physician. If you are in doubt about a driver's ability to navigate a vehicle safely, a formal driving evaluation may be advisable.

Other hazardous behaviors worthy of concern include possession of guns, home repair, and lawn mowers. Healthy people in the United States frequently have accidents with guns without having sensory changes with aging or cognitive impairment. The presence of cognitive impairment can certainly alter a person's ability to safely handle a firearm. Also, power tools such as lawn mowers may be dangerous machines if misused.

Trauma

The danger of cumulative and repetitive trauma to the brain has been known for many years. In the 1980s, scientists learned that head injuries double the risk of Alzheimer's disease.[175] In recent years, a dangerous, new result of head injury has been identified: chronic traumatic encephalopathy (CTE). This new condition is discussed in Chapter 7. Research led by Dr. Anne McKee and colleagues at Boston University has shown that both professional and college football players are at high risk for CTE.[78]

The human brain is not well protected from damages inflicted by physical forces. The best way to summarize the danger of head injuries is to say all injuries to the head are bad, including big ones and repetitive small ones. It is not only large injuries resulting in unconsciousness that are bad for the brain. The lingering effects of head injuries such as CTE include cognitive impairment, depression, irritability, loss of motor function, and, at times, suicide. CTE is currently untreatable and difficult to diagnose. It is reasonable to suggest that humans shouldn't participate in sports or activities associated with damage to the brain. It is certain that head injuries impair cognitive reserve and enhance the chance of cognitive losses with aging.

It is certain that head injuries impair cognitive reserve and enhance the chance of cognitive losses with aging.

A reasonable goal for all persons, young and old, is to avoid all head injuries, both big and small. There are many sports to choose from that have a low risk of head injury. A neurosurgeon colleague who is fond of American football, and an advisor to an National Football League team, once told me that contact sport "builds character." I don't deny that, but there are many ways to build character without irrevocably damaging the most delicate and critical part of one's body. Encourage your children and grandchildren to play sports with little risk of head injury.

The popularity of American football shows that the importance of brain health is not properly recognized. It is well known that small and large injuries to the head in American football damage the central nervous system and lead to serious consequences, as noted above. This lack of appreciation for the work of the brain may be because its contribution to our daily lives is largely invisible. We can't see how it's working. Of course, our experience of our daily lives is a manifestation of the brain's work, but this perspective is not widely appreciated. While visiting the United Kingdom, I saw a sticker on a motorcycle proclaiming, "Brain is Optional." I wish I'd had an opportunity to ask the motorcycle's owner about how he managed to ride without contributions from his brain.

While watching television one day, I stumbled upon the PBR channel. PBR is short for Professional Bull Riding. After climbing on top of an unhappy bull inside a pen, handlers open the pen and the bull darts into a dirt arena and begins bucking. The goal of the rider is to stay on top of the bull for eight seconds. Of course, at the end of eight seconds the bull does not stop to allow the rider to gently descend. Rather, the animal keeps working to send the rider to the ground.

Most of the riders wore cowboy hats, not helmets. Then I saw a rider with a helmet, and the announcer said, "It's good to see this rider back again. He had a head injury last year and has made the slow recovery but we're glad he's back on the bull. That's why he's wearing a helmet."

I found it hard to believe that I was hearing an apology for a bull rider to be wearing a helmet, as if it's not something any sane person should do while riding a bull. In any case, this bull had a novel movement that quickly smashed the rider's head into its horns. The rider lost consciousness and was hurtled to the ground. As he was taken off in a stretcher, the announcer said, "That's really too bad, that's not the kind of injury we like to see." What injury would they like to see? Well, that was left to the imagination.

Older people experience pathological changes to the spinal column in both the neck and the lumbar regions, as they age. This is produced by degenerative changes in the joints between the vertebrae in the neck and the lower spine with damage to cartilage. In most people, these changes do not cause serious symptoms or disability. However, some activities can cause problems to develop because of these age-related changes within the skeleton. Thus, older people should avoid carrying exceptionally heavy objects or lifting objects using their back instead of leg muscles.

Furthermore, important blood vessels travel through the cervical spine in the neck to reach the brain. Flow in these vessels is impaired by prolonged extension of the head, which is what happens when you tilt your head back and look up. These vessel changes can cause dizziness, vertigo (the sensation that the room or you is moving when it's not) and also fainting, falling, or strokes. Older people should not hold the head tilted back in this manner for longer than a few seconds. Activities to avoid include painting the ceiling, changing light bulbs, cleaning Venetian blinds, placing objects or retrieving objects from high shelves, using a ladder, and similar activities. Don't store your brown rice, dates, almonds, and whole wheat flour in a high cabinet requiring you to use a step stool to reach it.

Instead, store these items in a low cabinet that is easy to reach (hopefully frequently!).

Manipulations involving the neck can also cause blockage of the small important blood vessels that travel through the neck bones. For this reason, I recommend that chiropractic care be avoided because of the danger of damage to these vessels and potential stroke.[176]

25 TOXIC EXPOSURES

Because their multiple reserve factors are typically lower, older people are more sensitive to the toxic effects of environmental agents. The liver's ability to detoxify chemicals declines with age, as well as the ability of the kidney to excrete toxins. Everyone, especially the aged, should limit exposure to environmental toxins as much as possible, including air pollution, solvents, heavy metals, pesticides, herbicides, and other dangers. Exposure to toxins early in life may lower a person's physical reserve and result in cognitive impairment with aging. Exposure to pesticides and other toxins has been linked to Parkinson's disease.

Air pollution is also a risk factor for dementia. Particles in the air can enter the central nervous system through the olfactory nerves or through the blood–brain barrier and harm neurons and supporting cells. A study of 18,000 participants in the United States showed an association of air pollution with Alzheimer's pathology in the brain.[177] Considerable evidence shows that smoking increases the risk of cognitive impairment, stroke, and Alzheimer's disease, not to mention heart disease and cancer.[178] Toxic molecules can also be found in plastics. It is advisable to avoid microwaving food in plastic containers – glass is preferable.

In the 1980s, scientists wondered whether aluminum poisoning caused Alzheimer's disease. This proposal has been widely rejected. I saw a patient with motor neuron disease in the 1990s. He worked in a plant, pouring molten aluminum. A brain biopsy was done in order to measure the aluminum content in his brain. The biopsy was done with a plastic knife to diminish contamination of the brain specimen. These was no aluminum found in his brain, despite his high exposure.

The evolutionary aspects of toxins are of interest here. Lead is poisonous even in small doses, probably because it is present in very low amounts in the environment. Therefore, our ancestors didn't have the opportunity to develop ways to protect themselves from lead poisoning because they were not exposed. Aluminum, on the other hand, is the third most abundant molecule in the Earth's crust and the most abundant metal. However, it is highly toxic to the brain, and our ancestors, going back millions of years, had to develop effective ways to protect themselves from aluminum. Therefore, it is not necessary to replace aluminum pans in your kitchen.

Mercury is toxic to the brain and should certainly be avoided. However, there is no evidence that dental fillings containing mercury are hazardous to our health.

Alcohol

Excessive alcohol intake can damage several parts of your body and your physical reserve. It can also impair your cognitive reserve through impaired memory and learning. Alcohol abuse can lead to depression and poor psychological reserve, with loss of friends causing impaired social reserve.

What are the negative effects of alcohol on the body? It is a long and significant list, which includes, among others:

- direct toxicity to neurons,
- acutely and chronically diminished cognitive function,
- impaired balance and judgment,
- gastrointestinal bleeding,
- increased risk of intracranial hemorrhage,

- liver damage,
- injury to nerves in the leg and arms,
- injury to the cerebellum affecting walking and coordination,
- seizures,
- head injuries,
- trauma from falls and accidents,
- impairment of the immune system,
- colorectal cancer,
- altered absorption and metabolism of drugs, and
- decreased amount and quality of sleep.

An important consideration is that alcohol is metabolized largely by the liver and the function of that organ declines with age. A person who has been drinking 8 ounces a day of bourbon for many years and reaches the age of 80 may develop cognitive impairment from this amount of alcohol intake, even though he has been using it for many years without any negative effects. His 80-year-old liver may no longer be able to adequately metabolize alcohol and blood levels may have been rising as this lack of physical reserve developed. People who consume large amounts of alcohol or who are malnourished may be susceptible to thiamine (vitamin B1) and other vitamin deficiencies. This can cause acute onset of severe cognitive impairment, dizziness, visual changes, weakness, loss of consciousness, and death.

There are studies indicating that a moderate dose of alcohol may be protective against development of dementia with aging. But don't overdo it. It is important to be aware of how much you are drinking. People over the age of 60 shouldn't drink more than two doses of alcohol per day for men and one for women. One dose would be about 12 ounces of regular beer (about 5% alcohol), 5 ounces of wine (about 12% alcohol), or 1.5 ounces of distilled spirits (whisky, gin, bourbon, vodka, tequila, rum, about 40% alcohol). Remember that many wine glasses will not be filled halfway by 5 ounces of wine.

Studies show that more than one-third of drinkers over the age of 60 drink too much alcohol. Drinking too much on a daily basis is certainly to be avoided. It is also dangerous to consume too much on certain days (binge drinking). Beer and wine are not safer than other forms of alcohol – what is important is the dose of alcohol consumed.

Because of the general widespread negative effects of alcohol abuse, it's not recommended that people who do not drink should start drinking.

PART III

CONCLUSIONS

26 CONSIDERATIONS FOR SOCIETY AND THE FUTURE OF AGING

Worldwide Aging

Important global changes in the human aging are developing rapidly. Human life expectancy has doubled during the past century. Due to advances in public health, vaccines, and science, people are living longer. In Japan, in 2019, one in four of the population was aged over 65 years, marking a record high, and there are more elderly people than children. The Japanese bought 2.5 times more adult diapers than infant diapers in 2021. In the United Staes, 16 percent of the population are over the age of 65 and this percentage is expected to increase as people live longer and younger adults choose to have fewer children or no children at all.

The increase in the elderly population is happening in varying degrees all over the world. This expansion will cause enormous stress on global economies because of the need to support retired people, as well as the age-relatedness of diseases of the brain and body. Although heart disease and cancer rates are falling, Alzheimer's disease is increasing because of its strong link to aging and the lack of disease-modifying therapies. (People are living longer, which increases the number of people with Alzheimer's disease. The disease is decreasing if corrected for the increase in the number of people at risk, see Chapter 5.)

Public Policy and Aging

It is important to consider what can be done about the expansion of aged populations. The framework of the four reserve factors is a valuable way to envision responses. If every aged person were provided funds from the government to support education and activities to enhance development of cognitive, physical, psychological, and social reserves factors, healthcare costs would decrease significantly. Physical activities serve to enhance brain function as well as to reduce the risk of heart, lung, and other diseases associated with aging. Government policies to enhance prospects for physical and cognitive activities for older people are needed worldwide along with programs to enhance healthy diets. Community and political actions are needed to increase opportunities for mental and physical activity throughout life. Social engagement of older persons, including intergenerational relationships, must be facilitated.

A *forward-looking approach to healthcare will provide resources to people throughout life to keep them healthy and enhance their four reserve factors.*

A forward-looking approach to healthcare will provide resources to people throughout life to keep them healthy and enhance their four reserve factors. This is ethically and economically preferable to a healthcare system which only takes care of people when they're sick and doesn't strive to *prevent* illness. An excellent example is the value of education, which is protective against many illnesses. That is, people who are relatively more educated have a lower risk of Alzheimer's disease, heart disease, and many forms of cancer. Lifelong education has bountiful beneficial effects on health and healthcare expenses. It's also valuable to offer free public transportation to older people, which enhances their access to stimulating activities. In Japan, China, and the Netherlands, many older people use bicycles to get around with the assistance of bike lanes. Encouraging physical activity is an outstanding public health measure.

Public policy can improve diets with resultant improvement of the microbiota. Taxes and cost controls can enhance the consumption of whole-grain flour, brown rice, and other high-fiber foods (fruits, vegetables, legumes, nuts). Policies can also work to diminish the consumption of sugar, sodas, red meat, sports drinks, processed food, and fast food as well as artificial sugars, flavors, and colorings. Such policies will certainly be attacked in the United States as being a manifestation of government overreach. However, procedures are already in place in many regions to use the government to influence what people eat (examples include price supports, fortification of milk with vitamin D, import restrictions, Japanese government support of rice production, US support of corn). Why not go even further to promote healthy eating of fruits, vegetables, and the drinking of water, not soda? Government policies also influence pesticide exposures, as well as air and water pollution, which have negative influences on health and the microbiome, and enhance the risk of Alzheimer's disease. It's also helpful when restaurants make dietary information, including fiber content, available to customers.

As we have discussed, lifestyle factors influence health at all stages of life. Childhood is the best time to begin the beneficial habits of diet and exercise. Physical education should encourage children to participate in lifelong healthy sports such as running, walking, swimming, and tennis.[118] Many popular sports can't be played past middle age. Only eight in 10,000 high-school football players progress to the National Football League. Few people continue to play basketball into their 30s. The risk of head injury is another important matter (discussed in Chapter 7).

Personalized Medicine and Genetics

It is valuable for public health for persons to have the knowledge about their disease risks. The use of genetic information to assist in medical care has been called "personalized medicine" by Francis Collins, director of the US National Institutes of Health.[179] This is a valuable development with great promise. However, I object to the idea that personalized medicine requires genetic information. Personalized medicine is what every doctor should have been doing for the last several hundred years!

Physicians should know who the patient is in order to evaluate what's wrong and determine what the plan is for treatment.

Physicians should know who the patient is in order to evaluate what's wrong and determine what the plan is for treatment. Hippocrates said, "It is more important to know what sort of person has a disease than to know what sort of disease a person has." There are certainly times when genetic information helps. But knowledge of a patient's interests, capacities, and preferences is available now and is necessary for high-quality patient care.

Within the next 10 years, it's likely that sequencing of the entire genome of each patient will be routinely accomplished (whole-genome sequencing). The endeavor is called genomics. This will help with diagnosis, management, and evaluation of risks of disease. Genotype information can also help with understanding complexities of medication sensitivity and toxicity. Whole-genome sequencing will allow for an assessment of risk genes that have both large (such as apolipoprotein E, see Chapter 11) and small effects. This polygenic (multigene) risk hazard analysis may predict the occurrence of disease as well as the age of onset. The information provided by such a report will be hard for many people, including physicians, to comprehend.

It's worrisome that people are embarking on genetic testing that provides complex reports they can't understand. This is already true for many current genetic tests. Also, genetic testing may reveal evidence of a disease risk that can cause unnecessary anxiety. (This is also discussed in Chapter 11.) Education of the public and medical care providers about these developments is critical.

Genetic information that predicts the disease risk may help to motive people to eat better and to exercise. However, people at low genetic risk for Alzheimer's or Parkinson's diseases can still get either disease. Just because you're at low genetic risk doesn't mean you won't get the disease. Being a "couch potato" will definitely increase your risk of heart disease, stroke, Alzheimer's disease, Parkinson's disease, and other things.

Metagenomics

Information about the genetics of our microbes (metagenomics) will also be available to us in the near future. Science has shown us that every human is home to an ecosystem for countless microbial species. A new word has been coined to describe this ecosystem: a "holobiont," meaning the congregation of a host as well as other species living in and around it that together form a discrete biological unit. This amounts to a revolutionary change in our concept of the nature of our existence.

It may become routine that information about microbial DNA in the gut, including the mouth (the metagenome), will be tested. Similarly to whole-genome sequencing of a person's DNA, a report of the microbial DNA will be difficult to interpret by many people, including doctors. Abnormal microbiota in the mouth may be detected with a breath test, and urine tests for abnormal organic acids and assays for endotoxins (bacterial products) may help us understand the health of each person. Biotech companies are working on products designed to impact the production of trimethylamine by gut bacteria, to lower the risk of heart disease and perhaps Alzheimer's disease.[75] These therapeutic molecules as well as live bacteria (probiotics) are being designed to act only in the gut and not enter the bloodstream, so the risk of side effects should be low.

Drugs targeting human brain disease may derive therapeutic effects through their influence on the gut bacteria.

This approach to treatment and prevention of disease is revolutionary. Drugs targeting human brain disease may derive therapeutic effects through their influence on the gut bacteria. That is, new compounds for brain disorders may not need to enter the brain or cross the blood–brain barrier or enter the bloodstream. They may be effective through their actions on gut bacteria and their metabolites. A good example of this is the ability of polyphenols to inhibit amyloid aggregation in intestinal bacteria.[180] Fecal microbiota transplants are being developed with defined populations of bacteria, removing the need to use a human donor.[181]

Research is under way worldwide to develop precisely targeted populations of bacteria for use as probiotics. Also, prebiotic products to enhance the growth of helpful bacteria are being advanced and gut microbes are being studied as a source of drugs. Remember that many antibiotics are made by microorganisms, such as penicillin. The antibacterial actions of these microbial products are being studied as therapies for infectious diseases, in view of the rapid advance of antibiotic-resistant microbes worldwide.

As we have discussed, diet is key to health, not only because of the influence of diet on our bodies but because of its influence on our microbial inhabitants. It has been discovered that the effects of diet on our microbiota vary from person to person. Work is under way to develop personalized analytical methods to take this variation into account when giving dietary advice. It's likely that you'll soon be able to receive "personalized nutrition" advice, suited specifically to you.

Diagnosis

In recent years, there have been big advances in neuroimaging diagnosis of neurodegenerative diseases. Positron emission tomography (PET) scans can now detect signs of Alzheimer's disease using studies of glucose metabolism, cerebral blood flow, amyloid-beta and tau deposition, and white matter tract analysis. Early signs of Alzheimer's disease can now be detected 10 to 20 years before outward signs of the disease. Recent studies have shown a molecule in the blood from the brain of people with Alzheimer's disease that is highly specific and sensitive for the diagnosis.[182] Testing of similar molecules in the cerebral spinal fluid is also helpful. Another new development is skin biopsies, which are being used to detect Parkinson's disease.

An important issue in these studies is that the brain changes associated with these diseases can be detected many years before the first symptom. For example, about one-third of people over the age of 65 who are cognitively intact have a pattern of amyloid deposits in the brain associated with Alzheimer's disease.[183] This can now be detected through PET scanning. This may indicate that they will progress to develop dementia if they live long enough. However, we cannot determine when that will be and many persons with signs of Alzheimer's disease in the brain may die of other things before development of cognitive impairment. In the absence of an effective therapy, I question whether these tests are of clinical value, as they may cause unnecessary worry, and the recommended lifestyle actions are well known to be protective against heart disease and stroke. And even if genetic, blood tests, and brain imaging show that a person is at low risk of Alzheimer's disease, it is still important to have a healthy diet and exercise.

Consider a 70-year-old man with mild memory problems who has an amyloid PET scan showing the presence of amyloid deposits in the brain. This could be because the disease is beginning to establish itself in his brain and if he lives to be, say, 87 years old, he will develop cognitive impairment. However, most 70 year olds don't live to be 87, and it will be unfortunate if that person is told at the age of 70 that he has Alzheimer's disease and worries about it for the rest of his life but never develops dementia. The information from the scan or blood test may cause unnecessary stress. The reason for his memory problems at the age of 70 may be the result of something else entirely. Furthermore, most persons with signs of developing Alzheimer's disease in the brain who do not have cognitive impairment will die before they develop dementia.[60,183]

Furthermore, most persons with signs of developing Alzheimer's disease in the brain who do not have cognitive impairment will die before they develop dementia.

I believe the value of a diagnostic test is determined by whether it helps the patient or not. In the absence of a cure or really good treatment, the knowledge that a neurodegenerative process is under way may not have value and may, in fact, have negative consequences. This is especially true for people with the early signs of Alzheimer's disease found in the brain who will not live long enough to develop cognitive impairment. The situation will be different when there is a preventive or disease-modifying therapy. When that happens, it will be critical for presymptomatic testing to take place. so that people found to have signs in the brain for the disease can be properly treated. At the moment, such a treatment doesn't exist.

Artificial Intelligence

Due to great technological advances, artificial intelligence applications are already being developed for human health. Artificial intelligence is now being used as an aid to the interpretation of imaging studies. In some cases, it's been shown to be superior to the radiologist's assessment. Computer applications will be valuable in assisting the patient–doctor interaction. A network-linked camera in the office can evaluate a patient's speech, gait, and appearance, and may also help in diagnosis and disease management. Ideally, computer systems will be unified so that all of a patient's records will be available to every medical provider. I'd also like to see artificial intelligence developed to help physicians to be aware of a patient's activities, medication use, and diet.

In 2020, about 45 percent of the world's population owned smartphones. These phones and other wearable devices can be adapted to detect changes in voice, physical activities, and sleep cycles. Touch screens can assess motor function and can be adapted to measure heart function. Smartphones may help evaluate sleep, depression, and Parkinson's disease. A 2020 study used facial recognition technology to reliably identify political orientation.[184] If the technology can do that, it should be easier for software to assist doctors in diagnosis based on facial imaging and an evaluation of whole-body movement.

Enhancement of the four reserve factors can be aided by artificial intelligence.

Enhancement of the four reserve factors can be aided by artificial intelligence. It is already happening that interactions between humans and robots are becoming alternatives to human-to-human interactions. Robotic pets have been developed, such as a small stuffed toy dog that can be held in the lap and smile as it is patted. It will be critical for the developers of these devices and programs to appreciate the complexity of use for people with limited computer experience. Computer applications can also augment opportunities for social interactions of older people, aiding social reserve. The use of computers to develop friendships should not be limited to the young!

There has been an enormous advance in opportunities for interfaces of people with machines to provide complex cognitive stimulation, aiding cognitive reserve. These avenues are particularly important for older people with limited mobility. It will be critical that advances are made in the accessibility of these resources to people with limited mobility, sensory deficits, and cognitive impairment. Voice recognition software will be helpful to allow participants to access computer resources without knowing how to move a mouse or select a computer program.

Consider an activity room in a nursing home today. It's likely there are a group of residents sitting in chairs with a television broadcasting soap operas or game shows. This activity provides no opportunity for participation or interaction. Ideally, people working at the facility would know that one of the residents living there had been, for example, an oil painter and is able to provide an interactive visit for residents to the Portrait Gallery or the British Museum in London. Computer applications for the home, assisted-living facilities, and nursing homes can foster cognitive and physical stimulation that benefits all four of the reserve factors. However, the uses of technology must adapt to the special needs of the elderly. There is a long history of technology ignoring the need of people in this age group. For example, the size of letters in signs used in traffic control is based on the perceptual abilities of young people, not on the lower visual functioning of older drivers.

Artificial intelligence will also be of value in dealing with polypharmacy (the use of many medications by one person). Automated drug delivery systems can be provided to assist the patient in taking their medications at the right time, in the correct doses. This information can be forwarded through the internet to family members and medical professionals. Activity monitors can assess physical activity and forward data to caregivers and doctors.

It is hoped that advances in public policy and technology will help us to enhance our reserve factors and help us to avoid disease and remain fit as we age.

27 OUR ATTITUDE AND THE OPPORTUNITY OF AGING

Our greatest freedom is the freedom to choose our attitude.
Viktor Frankl, in *Man's Search for Meaning*

The word attitude has a variety of definitions. The Cambridge Dictionary defines it as "a way of behaving that is caused by a feeling or opinion about something or someone," while in the Oxford English Dictionary Online it is defined as a "deliberately adopted, or habitual, mode of regarding the object of thought." However we choose to define it, our attitude is something we carry around with us at all times. As the psychiatrist Victor Frankl said, we can choose how we approach life.

Our attitude is determined in large part by the focusing of our attention. If our attention is focused on losses and regrets, our attitude will be gloomy. If our attention is focused on opportunities, such as the opportunity of aging, our attitude will be more positive. This is a fundamental daily choice. It's necessary to appreciate that attention is the key to forming our attitude, not only experience. As noted in Chapter 15, William James asserted how attention determines how our experiences are managed by the brain, stating "My experience is what I agree to attend to."[135]

If our attention is focused on opportunities, such as the opportunity of aging, our attitude will be more positive. This is a fundamental daily choice.

The world we inhabit it too multifaceted for us to process all possible perceptions. It is our attention which is critical for the quality of our experience. And the focusing of our attention determines the quality of our outlook on life, our attitude.

The importance of attention to our attitude and our appreciation of life is illustrated by this question, "Why does time travel faster when we get older?" The perception of time is, of course, a neurological phenomenon, related to the sensory experiences of our daily lives. We cannot directly perceive the passage of time, as time is an abstraction. We do not perceive time; we perceive what goes on in time. Age-related declines in dopamine and other important neurotransmitters may produce the feeling that time travels faster as we get older.[185] It may also be that younger persons experience more novelty in daily life then older people. Each day is a smaller part of our life then previous days; one year is 10 percent of the life of a 10-year-old child, and 2 percent of the life of a 50-year-old adult. Consider what happens when we travel; in a new location we encounter novel stimuli, which require more processing than the ones we have become accustomed to. Stimuli that are not changing or that are long-standing do not attract our attention. It's not uncommon to feel that time is flying by when you are in a stable environment while on a trip you may have the impression that a week feels like a month.

The phenomenon that time travels faster when you get older is a reminder of the importance of novelty, diversity, and attention. If your daily life is consumed with watching reruns of television shows you have already seen, you are giving your nervous system few stimuli. But if you travel to a new place, you will encounter novelty. Travel is not the only way to experience novelty, of course. All learning is an exploration of novelty, and a diversity of experience enhances the resilience of the nervous system (cognitive reserve factor) as well as the resilience of the other reserve factors.

The use of the power of attention is essential. The brain has a dedicated system for the direction and intensity of attention, which involves the frontal lobes as well as evolutionarily ancient parts of the base of the brain, called the brainstem. However, all the four lobes of the cerebral cortex are involved in attention, not only the frontal lobes. Our attentional capacity is so great because it is imperative for our survival, now as well as the ancient past.

Our attitude is determined by the object of our attention. And our capacity of paying attention can be exercised and practiced every day, just as a pianist plays scales regularly to keep skills active. The brain is not good at multitasking and attention cannot be divided without a loss of quality. Presenting the brain with many undertakings at once leads to an inability to focus on anything at all. Multitasking is based on the fallacy that your brain can do two things well at the same time. It cannot. All that is possible is to switch back and forth quickly, impairing performance and creating the impression that you are doing two things at once. Proper attention is "single-minded." That is, if you are listening to someone speaking, simply listen. Do not prepare to speak as you listen. If you are going for a walk outside, experience the world through your attention. Don't occupy your mind with thoughts of regret, fear, and discontent. (And don't use earphones on your walk to listen to a discussion of the latest political scandal.) As William James once said, "The greatest weapon against stress is our ability to choose one thought over another."

Meditation is an excellent way to develop capacities for paying attention. Of course, it's possible to exercise our attentional capacities at every moment, not only while meditating. Paying attention is an intrinsically joyful experience. Mountain climbers risk their lives on dangerous avalanche-prone slopes because of the joy experienced by the intensity of their attention. The purposeful focusing of attention can lead to a state called "flow," resulting in the active experience of pleasure and meaning, according to psychologist Mihaly Csikszentmihalyi.[186] We have evolved the capacity to feel pain because it is a good warning that there is potential damage to the body. And we have evolved the capacity to experience joy when we pay attention because it helps us to survive. The joyful nature of attention helps us to do it well.

The joyful nature of attention helps us to do it well.

The focus of our attention must include ourselves, as well as the world. In James Joyce's *A Painful Case* (in the collection of short stories, *The Dubliners*, first published in 1914), he wrote that "Mr. Duffy lived a short distance from his body." Disconnection from the body can involve a detachment from one's feelings, thoughts, emotions, perceptions, and identity. Disconnection from our bodies causes disconnection from the world as well. There is a close relationship between emotion and the body.[1] Attention to ourselves, including the body, is critical.

Mountain climbers need not expose themselves to fatal falls because of their wish to experience the intense attention they find joyful. They could learn to practice this same feeling of the joy of attention in their everyday lives without the risk of death. Likewise, many people fail to appreciate opportunities to develop healthful attitudes about aging through the proper management of attention. Our multiple reserve factors and our ability to appreciate the opportunity of aging can be enhanced through attentiveness to the possibilities for enhancing our lives through actions.

---

[1] William James wrote extensively on this topic.[187]

I like the positive attitude suggested by the feminist author Christina Crosby. She wrote about her trauma-induced disability this way: "I am no longer what I once was – yet come to think of it, neither are you. All of us who live on are not what we were, but are becoming, always becoming."[188] What a critical realization, to acknowledge that we are all still becoming, always becoming, despite the challenges of aging.

This lifelong process of becoming is under our control. In the words of the philosopher Ralph Waldo Emerson, "A man is what he thinks about all day long." You could say that about aging. The quality of aging is related to what you think about all day long, what you pay attention to all day long, what your body is doing all day long, what you are eating all day long, what injuries you subject yourself to all day long; and how you are able to manage and enhance your cognitive, physical, psychological, and social reserve factors to attain and maintain health and fitness with age.

We must not presume aging to be inevitable and accept decline without consideration of how the manifestations of aging can be modified through our personal actions.

We must not presume aging to be inevitable and accept decline without consideration of how the manifestations of aging can be modified through our personal actions. Every moment we are alive is an occasion to experience the world and ourselves. Every moment is an occasion we should not allow to go by without notice.

Viewing aging as an opportunity helps to focus on the reality that what happens to us is determined in large part by what we do. Paying attention to what happens to us can enhance all of our reserve factors. Diet, physical and mental activities, and social and family contacts are all critical. Our enhancement of the four reserve factors will increase our chance to be healthy and fit as we age.

The word "opportunity" evolved from the Latin phrase "ob portum veniens," indicating a favorable wind coming to port, according to the Online Etymology Dictionary. We need to take advantage of all the favorable winds we have, especially those that help us to age well. The concept of the four reserve factors helps us to manage our sails so that we can gather the favorable winds and use them throughout our lifetime, to achieve and maintain the meaning of our lives.

We need to take advantage of all the favorable winds we have, especially those that help us to age well.

ACKNOWLEDGMENTS

The idea of this book originated in decades of discussions about aging with patients, families, friends, and relatives. It would not have been possible without the valuable assistance and support I have received from my wife, Shivani Nandi, who has been the center of my happiness every day of my life since 1999. Her encouragement and rational thinking have been critical for the book's progress and completion. I am also forever grateful for the love for learning that I acquired from my parents Gladys and Abraham Friedland, who taught me to think for myself. I stand in awe of my aunt Sophia Strong's indomitable spirit, who published a book at the age of 92 on her postwar travels in Japan and attended astrophysics classes at the age of 93.

I am appreciative for the wonderful mentorship I received from Morris B. Bender, who instilled in me the importance of listening to the patient, and Edwin A. Weinstein for teaching me the role of language in thought. I am also thankful and humbled by the exemplary and compassionate patient care of the many nurses and nurse practitioners I am fortunate to have worked with, especially Pamela Reichelt and Cathy Bays. A constant pillar of support and encouragement in my endeavors is Kerri Remmel, to whom I am deeply grateful. I'm indebted to Jignesh Shah, Demetra Antimisiaris, and Qi Dai for suggestions on earlier versions of the book.

I am also deeply grateful for the exceptional assistance of Anna Whiting, Zoë Lewin, and Ruth Boyes of Cambridge University Press and editor Todd Melby. The contributions of graphic designer Heather Jones are also acknowledged with thanks. My research work, which has provided me with the foundation of this book, would not have been possible without the support provided by the University of Louisville, the family of Edward A. Ford III, Walter Cowan, the V.V. Cooke Foundation, the Michael J. Fox Foundation for Parkinson's Research, the Mason and Mary Rudd family, the Kentucky Science and Engineering Foundation, and the Jewish Heritage Fund for Excellence.

GLOSSARY

aging: the process or condition of growing old.

cognition: "the action or faculty of knowing; knowledge, consciousness; acquaintance with a subject." (Oxford Engligh Dictionary Online)

delirium: a disorder of consciousness characterized by hallucinations, delusions, disorientation, impaired awareness, and often agitation; usually of abrupt onset.

delusions: fixed false beliefs, often of persecution (paranoia) or grandiosity, which are contrary to reality.

dementia: a clinical syndrome and not a specific disease, characterized by memory loss and other cognitive impairments, such as difficulty with route finding, language, perception, abstractions, calculations, behavior, spatial tasks, emotions, and reasoning. Dementia is usually, but not always, of slow onset.

dependence: "the situation in which you need something or someone all the time, especially in order to continue existing or operating." (The Cambridge Dictionary)

dysbiosis: an unhealthy population of microbes in the body, which may be caused by a lack of diversity or a gain or loss of members of the community.

epigenetics: the study of the modifications of the DNA in an organism that do not involve changes in the nucleotide sequence.

genomics: the study of genes. A genome is a complete set of all the DNA and the genes of an organism.

gerontology: the scientific study of the biological, social, psychological, and cognitive aspects of aging in animals and humans.

hallucinations: sensory experiences that appear to be real but are not. They can involve any of the five senses.

holobiont: a grouping comprised of a host and other species living inside and on its surface, forming a biological unit.

homeostasis: "the ability or tendency of a living organism, cell, or group to keep the conditions inside it the same despite any changes in the conditions around it, or the state of internal balance." (Cambridge Dictionary)

inflammaging: activation of the immune system seen with aging.

inflammation: the body's response to invasion by foreign organisms and its efforts to repair injury.

interdependence: "the fact of depending on each other." (Cambridge Dictionary)

magnetic resonance imaging (MRI): a medical imaging technique to produce images of the anatomy of the body, using strong magnetic fields and radio waves.

medication compliance: the extent to which a person follows the recommendations of a provider for the use of medications.

metagenomics: the study of the genetic information recovered from an environmental sample.

microbiome: the collective genome of our indigenous microbes.

microbiota: the microbial organisms that live inside us and on our body surfaces and cavities. They are comprised of bacteria, viruses, parasites, and fungi.

microglia: the major cells of the immune system in the brain that are responsible for maintaining homeostasis, monitoring the brain to defend against challenges.

misfolding: when a protein adopts an incorrect three-dimensional structure, which may prevent the protein from working and may make it have toxic effects.

neurodegenerative disease: a type of disease of the nervous system in which there is loss of cells and function. The disease is progressive after slow onset, may or may not be inherited, and may or may not have effective therapies. This includes Alzheimer's disease, Parkinson's disease, amyotrophic lateral sclerosis, and others.

pathogen: an agent which causes disease (such as smallpox).

pathogenesis: the process of initiation and maintenance of disease.

plasticity: the quality of being soft enough to be changed in to a new shape, the ability of a biological system to change.

polypharmacy: the regular use of five or more medications.

protein folding: the process through which a protein adopts a three-dimensional structure.

reserve: "to keep something for a particular purpose or time" (Cambridge Dictionary) (Latin: *reservare*, keep back, save up).

resilience: "the quality of being able to return quickly to a previous good condition after problems." (Cambridge Dictionary)

salutogenesis: to create health (Latin: *salus*, health, *genere*, to create).

symbiont: an organism living in symbiosis with another organism, in which each benefit.

symbiosis (or mutualism): an association between two organisms in which each benefit, such as birds that live near large animals who eat insects off of their hides.

tolerance: an active state where there is a lack of response to specific organisms or proteins in order to diminish potentially destructive immune responses. Also referred to as immune tolerance.

REFERENCES

1. Bernard C. *Lectures on the Phenomena of Life Common to Animals and Plants*. Charles C Thomas Publishing; 1974.
2. Franceschi C, Garagnani P, Parini P, Giuliani C, Santoro A. Inflammaging: a new immune-metabolic viewpoint for age-related diseases. *Nat Rev Endocrinol*. 2018;14(10):576–90.
3. Lorch M. Language and memory disorder in the case of Jonathan Swift: considerations on retrospective diagnosis. *Brain*. 2006;129(Pt 11):3127–37.
4. Antonovsky A. *Health, Stress and Coping*. Jossey-Bass Publishing; 1979.
5. Garmany A, Yamada S, Terzic A. Longevity leap: mind the healthspan gap. *NPJ Regen Med*. 2021;6(1):57.
6. North BJ, Sinclair DA. The intersection between aging and cardiovascular disease. *Circ Res*. 2012;110(8):1097–108.
7. Livingston G, Huntley J, Sommerlad A, et al. Dementia prevention, intervention, and care: 2020 report of the Lancet Commission. *Lancet*. 2020;396(10248):413–46.
8. Fratiglioni L, Marseglia A, Dekhtyar S. Ageing without dementia: can stimulating psychosocial and lifestyle experiences make a difference? Lancet Neurol. 2020;19(6):533–43.
9. Baker GT, Martin GR, Molecular and biologic factors in aging: the origins, causes, and prevention of senescence. In *Geriatric Medicine*, 3rd ed. Cassel CK , Cohen HJ, Larson LB, et al. (eds.), Springer Verlag; 1997, pp. 3–28,
10. Rowe JW, Kahn RL. Human aging: usual and successful. *Science*. 1987;237(4811):143–9.
11. Schott JM. The neurology of ageing: what is normal? *Pract Neurol*. 2017;17(3):172–82.

12. Soldan A, Pettigrew C, Albert M. Cognitive reserve from the perspective of preclinical Alzheimer disease: 2020 update. *Clin Geriatr Med*. 2020;36(2):247–63.

13. Klein RS. On complement, memory, and microglia. *N Engl J Med*. 2020;382(21):2056–8.

14. Baudisch A. *Inevitable Aging?: Contributions to Evolutionary-Demographic Theory*. Springer; 2008.

15. Barulli D, Stern Y. Efficiency, capacity, compensation, maintenance, plasticity: emerging concepts in cognitive reserve. *Trends Cogn Sci*. 2013;17(10):502–9.

16. Gonneaud J, Bedetti C, Pichet Binette A, et al. Association of education with Abeta burden in preclinical familial and sporadic Alzheimer disease. *Neurology*. 2020;95(11):e1554–64.

17. Friedland RP, Fritsch T, Smyth KA, et al. Patients with Alzheimer's disease have reduced activities in midlife compared with healthy control-group members. *Proc Natl Acad Sci U S A*. 2001;98(6):3440–5.

18. Mortimer JA, Borenstein AR, Gosche KM, Snowdon DA. Very early detection of Alzheimer neuropathology and the role of brain reserve in modifying its clinical expression. *J Geriatr Psychiatry Neurol*. 2005;18(4):218–23.

19. Ganz AB, Beker N, Hulsman M, et al. Neuropathology and cognitive performance in self-reported cognitively healthy centenarians. *Acta Neuropathol Commun*. 2018;6(1):64.

20. Snowdon D. *Aging with Grace: What the Nun Study Teaches Us about Leading Longer, Healthier, and More Meaningful Lives*. Bantam; 2002.

21. Snowdon DA, Greiner LH, Mortimer JA, et al. Brain infarction and the clinical expression of Alzheimer disease. The Nun Study. *JAMA*. 1997;277(10):813–7.

22. Oveisgharan S, Wilson RS, Yu L, Schneider JA, Bennett DA. Association of early-life cognitive enrichment with Alzheimer disease pathological changes and cognitive decline. *JAMA Neurol*. 2020;77(10):1217–24.

23. Pulido RS, Munji RN, Chan TC, et al. Neuronal activity regulates blood–brain barrier efflux transport through endothelial circadian genes. *Neuron*. 2020;108(5):937–52.e7.

24. Hobson P, Lewis A, Nair H, Wong S, Kumwenda M. How common are neurocognitive disorders in patients with chronic kidney disease and diabetes? Results from a cross-sectional study in a community cohort of patients in North Wales, UK. *BMJ Open*. 2018;8(12):e023520.

25. Evans IEM, Llewellyn DJ, Matthews FE, et al. Social isolation, cognitive reserve, and cognition in healthy older people. *PLoS One*. 2018;13(8):e0201008.

26. Dafsari FS, Jessen F. Depression: an underrecognized target for prevention of dementia in Alzheimer's disease. *Transl Psychiatry*. 2020;10(1):160.

27. Aizenstein HJ, Nebes RD, Saxton JA, et al. Frequent amyloid deposition without significant cognitive impairment among the elderly. *Arch Neurol*. 2008;65(11):1509–17.

28. Krystal H. *Integration and Self Healing: Affect, Trauma, Alexithymia*. The Analytic Press; 1988.

29. Erikson EH. *Identity and the Life Cycle*. W. W. Norton & Company; 1994.

30. Wilson RS, Krueger KR, Arnold SE, et al. Loneliness and risk of Alzheimer disease. *Arch Gen Psychiatry*. 2007;64(2):234–40.

31. Berry W. *Another Turn of the Crank: Essays*. Counterpoint; 1995.

32. Bennett DA, Schneider JA, Tang Y, Arnold SE, Wilson RS. The effect of social networks on the relation between Alzheimer's disease pathology and level of cognitive function in old people: a longitudinal cohort study. *Lancet Neurol*. 2006;5(5):406–12.

33. Wang HS. Dementia in old age. *Contemp Neurol Ser*. 1977;15:15–27.

34. Friedland RP, Nandi S. A modest proposal for a longitudinal study of dementia prevention (with apologies to Jonathan Swift, 1729). *J Alzheimers Dis*. 2013;33(2):313–5.

35. Cobb M. *The Idea of the Brain: The Past and Future of Neuroscience*. Basic Books; 2020.

36. Fine I, Park JM. Blindness and human brain plasticity. *Annu Rev Vis Sci*. 2018;4:337–56.

37. Maguire EA, Nannery R, Spiers HJ. Navigation around London by a taxi driver with bilateral hippocampal lesions. *Brain*. 2006;129(Pt 11):2894–907.

38. Yong E. *How Brain Scientists Forgot That Brains Have Owners*. The Atlantic; 2017.

39. Bennett J. *On Human Origins, Spirituality and the Meaning of Life*. Friesen Press; 2021, p. 235.

40. Schulte BPM. John Hughlings Jackson. In Eling P (ed.), *Reader in the History of Aphasia*. Benjamins; 1994, pp. 133–67.

41. Jackson JH. *BMJ*. 1884;I:662.

42. Badimon A, Strasburger HJ, Ayata P, et al. Negative feedback control of neuronal activity by microglia. *Nature*. 2020;586(7829):417–23.

43. Buffington SA, Di Prisco GV, Auchtung TA, et al. Microbial reconstitution reverses maternal diet-induced social and synaptic deficits in offspring. *Cell*. 2016;165(7):1762–75.

44. Li Q, Barres BA. Microglia and macrophages in brain homeostasis and disease. *Nat Rev Immunol*. 2018;18(4):225–42.

45. Vuong HE, Pronovost GN, Williams DW, et al. The maternal microbiome modulates fetal neurodevelopment in mice. *Nature*. 2020;586(7828):281–6.

46. Strittmatter A, Sunde U, Zegners D. Life cycle patterns of cognitive performance over the long run. *Proc Natl Acad Sci U S A*. 2020;117(44):27255–61.

47. Davidow Hirshbein L. William Osler and The Fixed Period: conflicting medical and popular ideas about old age. *Arch Intern Med*. 2001;161(17):2074–8.

48. Gravitz L. The forgotten part of memory. *Nature*. 2019;571(7766):S12–S14.

49. Fishman E. Risk of developing dementia at older ages in the United States. *Demography*. 2017;54(5):1897–919.

50. Association Association. Alzheimer's disease facts and figures. Alzheimer's Association Report. Alzheimer's Association, March 10, 2020. doi: https://doi.org/10.1002/alz.12068.

51. Kalaria RN, Maestre GE, Arizaga R, et al. Alzheimer's disease and vascular dementia in developing countries: prevalence, management, and risk factors. Lancet Neurol. 2008;7(9):812–26.

52. Barnes LL. Alzheimer disease in African American individuals: increased incidence or not enough data? Nat Rev Neurol. 2022;18(1):56–62.

53. Engstrom EJ, Burgmair W, Weber MM. Emil Kraepelin's "self-assessment": clinical autography in historical context. Hist Psychiatry. 2002;13(49 Pt 1): 89–119.

54. Freyhan FA, Woodford RB, Kety SS. Cerebral blood flow and metabolism in psychoses of senility. J Nerv Ment Dis. 1951;113(5):449–56.

55. Katzman R. Editorial: The prevalence and malignancy of Alzheimer disease. A major killer. Arch Neurol. 1976;33(4): 217–8.

56. Friedland RP, Chapman MR. The role of microbial amyloid in neurodegeneration. PLoS Pathog. 2017;13(12):e1006654.

57. Friedland RP. Mechanisms of molecular mimicry involving the microbiota in neurodegeneration. J Alzheimers Dis. 2015;45(2):349–62.

58. Ayres JS. The biology of physiological health. Cell. 2020;181(2):250–69.

59. Ayres JS, Schneider DS. Tolerance of infections. Annu Rev Immunol. 2012;30:271–94.

60. Espay A, Stecher B. Brain Fables: The Hidden History of Neurodegenerative Diseases and a Blueprint to Conquer Them. Cambridge University Press; 2020, pp. 111–23.

61. Levine DA, Gross AL, Briceno EM, et al. Association between blood pressure and later-life cognition among black and white individuals. JAMA Neurol. 2020;77(7):810–9.

62. Frisoni GB, Molinuevo JL, Altomare D, et al. Precision prevention of Alzheimer's and other dementias: anticipating future needs in the control of risk factors and implementation of disease-modifying therapies. *Alzheimers Dement*. 2020;16(10):1457–68.

63. Xu W, Tan L, Wang HF, et al. Education and risk of dementia: dose-response meta-analysis of prospective cohort studies. *Mol Neurobiol*. 2016;53(5):3113–23.

64. Fink HA, Linskens EJ, MacDonald R, et al. Benefits and harms of prescription drugs and supplements for treatment of clinical Alzheimer-type dementia. *Ann Intern Med*. 2020;172(10):656–68.

65. Kurlawala Z, Roberts JA, McMillan JD, Friedland RP. Diazepam toxicity presenting as a dementia disorder. *J Alzheimers Dis*. 2018;66(3):935–8.

66. Friedland RP. "Normal"-pressure hydrocephalus and the saga of the treatable dementias. *JAMA*. 1989;262(18): 2577–81.

67. Ohnmacht J, May P, Sinkkonen L, Kruger R. Missing heritability in Parkinson's disease: the emerging role of non-coding genetic variation. *J Neural Transm (Vienna)*. 2020;127(5):729–48.

68. Kummer BR, Diaz I, Wu X, et al. Associations between cerebrovascular risk factors and Parkinson disease. *Ann Neurol*. 2019;86(4):572–81.

69. Ingre C, Roos PM, Piehl F, Kamel F, Fang F. Risk factors for amyotrophic lateral sclerosis. *Clin Epidemiol*. 2015;7: 181–93.

70. Einstein A. On the Method of Theoretical Physics. Lecture delivered at Oxford, June 10, 1933.

71. Gorelick PB, Scuteri A, Black SE, et al. Vascular contributions to cognitive impairment and dementia: a statement for healthcare professionals from the American Heart Association/American Stroke Association. *Stroke*. 2011;42(9):2672–713.

72. Gu Y, Gutierrez J, Meier IB, et al. Circulating inflammatory biomarkers are related to cerebrovascular disease in older adults. *Neurol Neuroimmunol Neuroinflamm*. 2019;6(1):e521.

73. Tonomura S, Ihara M, Kawano T, et al. Intracerebral hemorrhage and deep microbleeds associated with cnm-positive *Streptococcus mutans*: a hospital cohort study. *Sci Rep*. 2016;6:20074.

74. Tonomura S, Ihara M, Friedland RP. Microbiota in cerebrovascular disease: a key player and future therapeutic target. *J Cereb Blood Flow Metab*. 2020;40(7):1368–80.

75. Tang WH, Wang Z, Levison BS, et al. Intestinal microbial metabolism of phosphatidylcholine and cardiovascular risk. *N Engl J Med*. 2013;368(17):1575–84.

76. Gajdusek DC, Gibbs CJ, Alpers M. Experimental transmission of a kuru-like syndrome to chimpanzees. *Nature*. 1966;209(5025):794–6.

77. Friedland RP, Petersen RB, Rubenstein R. Bovine spongiform encephalopathy and aquaculture. *J Alzheimers Dis*. 2009;17(2):277–9.

78. Stern RA, Riley DO, Daneshvar DH, et al. Long-term consequences of repetitive brain trauma: chronic traumatic encephalopathy. 2011;3(10 Suppl 2):S460–7.

79. Darwin C, *Origin of Species*, second British edition; 1860, p. 3.

80. Leshem A, Liwinski T, Elinav E. Immune-microbiota interplay and colonization resistance in infection. *Mol Cell*. 2020;78(4):597–613.

81. Differding MK, Mueller NT. Human milk bacteria: seeding the infant gut? *Cell Host Microbe*. 2020;28(2):151–3.

82. Liu Q, Liu Q, Meng H, et al. *Staphylococcus epidermidis* contributes to healthy maturation of the nasal microbiome by stimulating antimicrobial peptide production. *Cell Host Microbe*. 2020;27(1):68–78 e5.

83. Faraco G, Hochrainer K, Segarra SG, et al. Dietary salt promotes cognitive impairment through tau phosphorylation. *Nature*. 2019;574(7780):686–90.

84. Kimura I, Miyamoto J, Ohue-Kitano R, et al. Maternal gut microbiota in pregnancy influences offspring metabolic phenotype in mice. *Science*. 2020;367(6481): eaaw8429.

85. D'Aquila P, Carelli LL, De Rango F, Passarino G, Bellizzi D. Gut microbiota as important mediator between diet and DNA methylation and histone modifications in the host. *Nutrients*. 2020;12(3):597.

86. Finlay BB, CFIR Humans & the Microbiome: Are noncommunicable diseases communicable? *Science*. 2020;367(6475):250–1.

87. Glowacki RWP, Martens EC. In sickness and health: effects of gut microbial metabolites on human physiology. *PLoS Pathog*. 2020;16(4):e1008370.

88. Itzhaki RF. A turning point in Alzheimer's disease: microbes matter. *J Alzheimers Dis*. 2019;72(4):977–80.

89. Dominy SS, Lynch C, Ermini F, et al. Porphyromonas gingivalis in Alzheimer's disease brains: evidence for disease causation and treatment with small-molecule inhibitors. *Sci Adv*. 2019;5(1):eaau3333.

90. O'Keefe SJ, Li JV, Lahti L, et al. Fat, fibre and cancer risk in African Americans and rural Africans. *Nat Commun*. 2015;6:6342.

91. Kohler W. *Dynamics in Psychology, Retention and Recall*. Liveright Publishing Corp.; 1940, pp. 115–6.

92. Friedland RP, McMillan JD, Kurlawala Z. What are the molecular mechanisms by which functional bacterial amyloids influence amyloid beta deposition and neuroinflammation in neurodegenerative disorders? *Int J Mol Sci*. 2020;21(5):1652.

93. Kowalski K, Mulak A. Brain–gut–microbiota axis in Alzheimer's disease. *J Neurogastroenterol Motil*. 2019;25(1): 48–60.

94. Kim S, Kwon SH, Kam TI, et al. Transneuronal propagation of pathologic α-synuclein from the gut to the brain models Parkinson's disease. *Neuron*. 2019;103(4):627–641.e7.

95. Xue QL. The frailty syndrome: definition and natural history. *Clin Geriatr Med*. 2011;27(1):1–15.

96. Claesson MJ, Jeffery IB, Conde S, et al. Gut microbiota composition correlates with diet and health in the elderly. *Nature*. 2012;488(7410):178–84.

97. Friedland RP, Haribabu B. The role for the metagenome in the pathogenesis of COVID-19. *EBioMedicine*. 2020;61:103019.

98. Alexander M, Turnbaugh PJ. Deconstructing mechanisms of diet–microbiome–immune interactions. *Immunity*. 2020;53(2):264–76.

99. Wene-Batu P, Bisimwa G, Baguma M, et al. Long-term effects of severe acute malnutrition during childhood on adult cognitive, academic and behavioural development in African fragile countries: the Lwiro cohort study in Democratic Republic of the Congo. *PLoS One*. 2020;15(12):e0244486.

100. Slade K, Plack CJ, Nuttall HE. The effects of age-related hearing loss on the brain and cognitive function. *Trends Neurosci*. 2020;43(10):810–21.

101. Knopman DS, Roberts RO. Healthy young hearts sharper older minds make. *Ann Neurol*. 2013;73(2):151–2.

102. Llewellyn DJ, Langa KM, Friedland RP, Lang IA. Serum albumin concentration and cognitive impairment. *Curr Alzheimer Res*. 2010;7(1):91–6.

103. Chrischilles E, Schneider K, Wilwert J, et al. Beyond comorbidity: expanding the definition and measurement of complexity among older adults using administrative claims data. *Med Care*. 2014;52(Suppl 3):S75–84.

104. Nesse RM. *Why We Get Sick: The New Science of Darwinian Medicine*. Vintage; 1996.

105. Lasselin J. Back to the future of psychoneuroimmunology: studying inflammation-induced sickness behavior. *Brain Behav Immun Health*. 2021;18:100379.

106. Song H, Sieurin J, Wirdefeldt K, et al. Association of stress-related disorders with subsequent neurodegenerative diseases. *JAMA Neurol*. 2020;77(6):700–9.

107. Krystal H. The aging survivor of the holocaust. Integration and self-healing in posttraumatic states. *J Geriatr Psychiatry*. 1981;14(2):165–89.

108. Zhou XL, Wang LN, Wang J, Shen XH, Zhao X. Effects of exercise interventions for specific cognitive domains in old adults with mild cognitive impairment: a protocol of subgroup meta-analysis of randomized controlled trials. *Medicine (Baltimore)*. 2018;97(48):e13244.

109. Bissell MJ. Asking the question of why. *Cell*. 2020;181(3): 503–6.

110. Farrer LA, Cupples LA, Haines JL, et al. Effects of age, sex, and ethnicity on the association between apolipoprotein E genotype and Alzheimer disease. A meta-analysis. APOE and Alzheimer Disease Meta Analysis Consortium. *JAMA*. 1997;278(16):1349–56.

111. Scheltens P, Blennow K, Breteler MM, et al. Alzheimer's disease. *Lancet*. 2016;388(10043):505–17.

112. Tran TTT, Corsini S, Kellingray L, et al. APOE genotype influences the gut microbiome structure and function in humans and mice: relevance for Alzheimer's disease pathophysiology. *FASEB J*. 2019;33(7):8221–31.

113. Konijnenberg E, Tomassen J, den Braber A, et al. Onset of preclinical Alzheimer disease in monozygotic twins. *Ann Neurol*. 2021;89(5):987–1000.

114. Daviglus ML, Bell CC, Berrettini W, et al. NIH State-of-the-Science Conference statement: preventing Alzheimer's disease and cognitive decline. *NIH Consens State Sci Statements*. 2010;27(4):1–30.

115. Daviglus ML, Plassman BL, Pirzada A, et al. Risk factors and preventive interventions for Alzheimer disease: state of the science. *Arch Neurol*. 2011;68(9):1185–90.

116. National Academies of Sciences, Engineering, and Medicine; Health and Medicine Division; Board on Health Sciences Policy; Committee on Preventing Dementia and Cognitive Impairment. *Preventing Cognitive Decline and Dementia: A Way Forward.* Downey A, Stroud C, Landis S, Leshner AI (eds.), National Academies Press; 2017.

117. Yu JT, Xu W, Tan CC, et al. Evidence-based prevention of Alzheimer's disease: systematic review and meta-analysis of 243 observational prospective studies and 153 randomised controlled trials. *J Neurol Neurosurg Psychiatry.* 2020; 91(11):1201–9.

118. Friedland RP, Brayne C. What does the pediatrician need to know about Alzheimer disease? *J Dev Behav Pediatr.* 2009;30(3):239–41.

119. Hurley D. Grandma's experiences leave a mark on your genes. *Discover.* 2015; June 25.

120. Gilbert J, Knight R. *Dirt Is Good: The Advantage of Germs for Your Child's Developing Immune System.* St. Martin's Press; 2017.

121. Norton S, Matthews FE, Barnes DE, Yaffe K, Brayne C. Potential for primary prevention of Alzheimer's disease: an analysis of population-based data. *Lancet Neurol.* 2014;13(8):788–94.

122. Kovari E, Herrmann FR, Bouras C, Gold G. Amyloid deposition is decreasing in aging brains: an autopsy study of 1,599 older people. *Neurology.* 2014;82(4):326–31.

123. Wu YT, Beiser AS, Breteler MMB, et al. The changing prevalence and incidence of dementia over time: current evidence. *Nat Rev Neurol.* 2017;13(6):327–39.

124. United States Census Bureau. Current Population Survey (CPS). 2021; December 14.

125. Krell-Roesch J, Syrjanen JA, Bezold J, et al. Physical activity and trajectory of cognitive change in older persons: Mayo Clinic Study of Aging. *J Alzheimers Dis.* 2021;79(1): 377–88.

126. Wilson EO. *Biophilia*. Harvard University Press; 1984.

127. Borenstein A, Mortimer J. *Alzheimer's Disease: Life Course Perspectives on Risk Reduction*. Academic Press; 2016.

128. Jung MS, Chung E. Television viewing and cognitive dysfunction of Korean older adults. *Healthcare (Basel)*. 2020;8(4):547.

129. Kehler DS, Hay JL, Stammers AN, et al. A systematic review of the association between sedentary behaviors with frailty. *Exp Gerontol*. 2018;114:1–12.

130. Takagi H, Hari Y, Nakashima K, Kuno T, Ando T, Group A. Meta-analysis of the relation of television-viewing time and cardiovascular disease. *Am J Cardiol*. 2019;124(11): 1674–83.

131. Gallucci M, Mazzarolo AP, Focella L, et al. 'Camminando e leggendo … "Ricordo" (walking and reading … I remember): prevention of frailty through the promotion of physical activity and reading in people with mild cognitive impairment. Results from the TREDEM Registry. *J Alzheimers Dis*. 2020;77(2):689–99.

132. Smyth KA, Fritsch T, Cook TB, et al. Worker functions and traits associated with occupations and the development of AD. *Neurology*. 2004;63(3):498–503.

133. Budson AE, O'Connor MK. *Seven Steps to Managing Your Memory: What's Normal, What's Not, and What to Do About It*. Oxford University Press; 2017.

134. Kornfield J. *A Path with Heart: A Guide through the Perils and Promises of Spiritual Life*. Bantam; 1993.

135. James W. *The Selected Letters of William James*. Anchor Books; 1993.

136. Schanche E, Vollestad J, Visted E, et al. The effects of mindfulness-based cognitive therapy on risk and protective factors of depressive relapse: a randomized wait-list controlled trial. *BMC Psychol*. 2020;8(1):57.

137. Barusch AS. *Love Stories of Later Life: A Narrative Approach to Understanding Romance*. Oxford University Press; 2008.

138. Gunak MM, Billings J, Carratu E, et al. Post-traumatic stress disorder as a risk factor for dementia: systematic review and meta-analysis. *Br J Psychiatry*. 2020;217(5):600–8.

139. Barthelemy NR, Liu H, Lu W, et al. Sleep deprivation affects tau phosphorylation in human cerebrospinal fluid. *Ann Neurol*. 2020;87(5):700–9.

140. Cascella M, Bimonte S, Barbieri A, et al. Dissecting the mechanisms and molecules underlying the potential carcinogenicity of red and processed meat in colorectal cancer (CRC): an overview on the current state of knowledge. *Infect Agent Cancer*. 2018;13:3.

141. Aune D, Keum N, Giovannucci E, et al. Whole grain consumption and risk of cardiovascular disease, cancer, and all cause and cause specific mortality: systematic review and dose–response meta-analysis of prospective studies. *BMJ*. 2016;353:i2716.

142. School of Public Health UoW. The Anti-Inflammatory Lifestyle. School of Medicine and Public Health, University of Wisconsin-Madison, 2018, p. 12.

143. Enders G. *Gut: The Inside Story of Our Body's Most Underrated Organ*. Greystone Books; 2018.

144. Shaikh FY, Sears CL. Messengers from the microbiota. *Science*. 2020;369(6510):1427–8.

145. Swaminathan S, Dehghan M, Raj JM, et al. Associations of cereal grains intake with cardiovascular disease and mortality across 21 countries in Prospective Urban and Rural Epidemiology study: prospective cohort study. *BMJ*. 2021;372:m4948.

146. Glenn AJ, Lo K, Jenkins DJA, et al. Relationship between a plant-based dietary portfolio and risk of cardiovascular disease: findings from the Women's Health Initiative Prospective Cohort Study. *J Am Heart Assoc*. 2021;10(16):e021515.

147. Kaplan A, Zelicha H, Meir AY, et al. The effect of a high-polyphenol Mediterranean diet (GREEN-MED) combined with

physical activity on age-related brain atrophy: the DIRECT
PLUS randomized controlled trial. *Am J Clin Nutr.* 2022.
doi: 10.1093/ajcn/nqac001.

148. Keenan TD, Agron E, Mares JA, et al. Adherence to a
Mediterranean diet and cognitive function in the Age-Related
Eye Disease Studies 1 & 2. *Alzheimers Dement.* 2020;16(6):831–42.

149. Harari Y. *Homo Deus: A Brief History of Tomorrow.* Harper; 2017.

150. Yin J, Zhu Y, Malik V, et al. Intake of sugar-sweetened and
low-calorie sweetened beverages and risk of cardiovascular
disease: a meta-analysis and systematic review. *Adv Nutr.*
2021;12(1):89–101.

151. Chong CP, Shahar S, Haron H, Din NC. Habitual sugar intake
and cognitive impairment among multi-ethnic Malaysian
older adults. *Clin Interv Aging.* 2019;14:1331–42.

152. United Brain Association. How sugar affects the brain.
Available from: https://unitedbrainassociation.org/2020/06/28/
how-sugar-affects-the-brain/.

153. Charisis S, Ntanasi E, Yannakoulia M, et al. Diet inflammatory
index and dementia incidence: a population-based study.
Neurology. 2021;97(24):e2381–91.

154. Shishtar E, Rogers GT, Blumberg JB, Au R, Jacques PF. Long-
term dietary flavonoid intake and risk of Alzheimer disease
and related dementias in the Framingham Offspring Cohort.
Am J Clin Nutr. 2020;112(2):343–53.

155. Neelakantan N, Seah JYH, van Dam RM. The effect of coconut
oil consumption on cardiovascular risk factors: a systematic
review and meta-analysis of clinical trials. *Circulation.*
2020;141(10):803–14.

156. Seshadri S, Beiser A, Selhub J, et al. Plasma homocysteine as a
risk factor for dementia and Alzheimer's disease. *N Engl J Med.*
2002;346(7):476–83.

157. Blacher E, Bashiardes S, Shapiro H, et al. Potential roles of
gut microbiome and metabolites in modulating ALS in mice.
Nature. 2019;572(7770):474–80.

158. Green KN, Steffan JS, Martinez-Coria H, et al. Nicotinamide restores cognition in Alzheimer's disease transgenic mice via a mechanism involving sirtuin inhibition and selective reduction of Thr231-phosphotau. *J Neuro*sci. 2008;28(45):11500–10.

159. Liebler DC. The role of metabolism in the antioxidant function of vitamin E. *Crit Rev Toxicol.* 1993;23(2):147–69.

160. Chen F, Du M, Blumberg JB, et al. Association among dietary supplement use, nutrient intake, and mortality among US adults: a cohort study. *Ann Intern Med.* 2019;170(9):604–13.

161. Kirichenko TV, Sukhorukov VN, Markin AM, et al. Medicinal plants as a potential and successful treatment option in the context of atherosclerosis. *Front Pharmacol.* 2020;11:403.

162. Fiala M, Liu PT, Espinosa-Jeffrey A, et al. Innate immunity and transcription of MGAT-III and Toll-like receptors in Alzheimer's disease patients are improved by bisdemethoxycurcumin. *Proc Natl Acad Sci U S A.* 2007;104(31):12849–54.

163. Yamasaki TR, Ono K, Ho L, Pasinetti GM. Gut microbiome-modified polyphenolic compounds inhibit alpha-synuclein seeding and spreading in alpha-synucleinopathies. *Front Neurosci.* 2020;14:398.

164. Noguchi-Shinohara M, Yuki S, Dohmoto C, et al. Consumption of green tea, but not black tea or coffee, is associated with reduced risk of cognitive decline. *PLoS One.* 2014;9(5):e96013.

165. Holland TM, Agarwal P, Wang Y, et al. Dietary flavonols and risk of Alzheimer dementia. *Neurology.* 2020;94(16):e1749–56.

166. de Cabo R, Mattson MP. Effects of intermittent fasting on health, aging, and disease. *N Engl J Med.* 2019;381(26): 2541–51.

167. Metchnikoff E. On the present state of the question of immunity and infectious diseases, Nobel Lecture, December 11, 1908.

168. Shah J. *Heart Health: A Guide to the Tests and Treatments You Really Need*. Rowman & Littlefield Publishers; 2019.

169. Friedland RP, Lerner AJ, Hedera P, Brass EP. Encephalopathy associated with bismuth subgallate therapy. *Clin Neuropharmacol*. 1993;16(2):173–6.

170. Maher RL, Hanlon J, Hajjar ER. Clinical consequences of polypharmacy in elderly. *Expert Opin Drug Saf*. 2014;13(1): 57–65.

171. Wastesson JW, Morin L, Tan ECK, Johnell K. An update on the clinical consequences of polypharmacy in older adults: a narrative review. *Expert Opin Drug Saf*. 2018;17(12):1185–96.

172. Chew ML, Mulsant BH, Pollock BG, et al. Anticholinergic activity of 107 medications commonly used by older adults. *J Am Geriatr Soc*. 2008;56(7):1333–41.

173. de Ropp RS. *The New Prometheans*. Delacorte; 1972, p. 80.

174. Brauer CA, Coca-Perraillon M, Cutler DM, Rosen AB. Incidence and mortality of hip fractures in the United States. *JAMA*. 2009;302(14):1573–9.

175. Fleminger S, Oliver DL, Lovestone S, Rabe-Hesketh S, Giora A. Head injury as a risk factor for Alzheimer's disease: the evidence 10 years on; a partial replication. *J Neurol Neurosurg Psychiatry*. 2003;74(7):857–62.

176. Harvard Health Publishing. Chiropractic neck adjustments linked to stroke. Available from: www.health.harvard.edu/ heart-health/chiropractic-neck-adjustments-linked-to-stroke.

177. Iaccarino L, La Joie R, Lesman-Segev OH, et al. Association between ambient air pollution and amyloid positron emission tomography positivity in older adults with cognitive impairment. *JAMA Neurol*. 2021;78(2):197–207.

178. Niu H, Qu Y, Li Z, et al. Smoking and risk for Alzheimer disease: a meta-analysis based on both case–control and cohort study. *J Nerv Ment Dis*. 2018;206(9):680–5.

179. Hamburg MA, Collins FS. The path to personalized medicine. *N Engl J Med*. 2010; 363(4):301–4. Erratum in *N Engl J Med*. 2010; 363(11):1092.

180. Sampson TR, Challis C, Jain N, et al. A gut bacterial amyloid promotes alpha-synuclein aggregation and motor impairment in mice. *Elife*. 2020;9:e53111.

181. Wargo JA. Modulating gut microbes. *Science*. 2020;369(6509):1302–3.

182. Palmqvist S, Tideman P, Cullen N, et al. Prediction of future Alzheimer's disease dementia using plasma phospho-tau combined with other accessible measures. *Nat Med*. 2021; 27(6):1034–42.

183. Brookmeyer R, Abdalla N. Estimation of lifetime risks of Alzheimer's disease dementia using biomarkers for preclinical disease. *Alzheimers Dement*. 2018;14(8):981–8.

184. Kosinski M. Facial recognition technology can expose political orientation from naturalistic facial images. *Sci Rep*. 2021;11(1):100. Erratum in *Sci Rep*. 2021;11(1):23228.

185. Efron R. The duration of the present. *Ann NY Acad Sci*. 1967;138(2):713–29.

186. Csikszentmihalyi M. *Flow: The Psychology of Optimal Experience*. Harper Perennial Modern Classics; 2008.

187. James W. What is an emotion? *Mind*. 1884:188–205.

188. Seelye KQ. Christina Crosby, 67, dies; feminist scholar wrote of becoming disabled. *NY Times*. 2021; January 26.

INDEX

acetylcholine, 260
acetylcholinesterase inhibitors, 103
adaptability, 45, 46, 47–51
adaptive immunity, 17, 88, 139
additives, 234, 235
aducanumab, 95
African Americans, 78, 112, 136, 138
aging, 4–16
  attitude to, 10, 292–7
  cognitive function and, 63
  drug interactions and, 261
  evolution and, 19–24
  immune systems in, 16–19
  mental health and, 166–7
  opportunity of, 5, 11, 296
  public policy and, 41, 282–3
  worldwide, 281
air pollution, 274, 283
albumin, 158
alcohol, 124, 172, 275–7
alpha synuclein, 101, 102
Alzheimer, Alois, 81
Alzheimer's disease, 3, 29, 76–84, 105
  brain and, 28, 84–6, 90
  case studies, 41, 75
  clinical trials, 266
  depression and, 34
  early onset, 174
  education and, 26
  four critical factors, 188–91
  inflammation in, 88
  memory loss, 67
  multiple reserves and, 39
  PET diagnosis, 287
  preventive measures, 185–8
  protein deposits and folding, 86–9
  research on, 265
  risk and protective factors, 93, 188
  sleep problems, 222
  smoking and, 33
  social isolation and, 36
  stroke and, 112
  treatments for, 94
  world patterns of, 135, 136
American football, 121, 270
amino acids, 86
amnesia, 69
amyloid precursor protein, 85
amyloids, 28, 85, 86, 87, 140, 287
amyotrophic lateral sclerosis (ALS), 99, 103–4, 105, 143, 179
anemia, 157
animal testing, 267
antibiotics, 286
anticholinergics, 260
antidepressants, 95, 168
anti-inflammatory state, 17, 18

antioxidants, 235, 241
APOE gene, 170–1, 174–81
artificial intelligence, 268, 289–91
atherosclerosis, 108
atrial fibrillation, 112, 157
atrophy, 85, 86, 99, 124, 172
attention, 69, 74, 203, 204, 292–7
attitude, 10, 292–7
auditory cortex, 57
auditory hallucinations, 63
autism spectrum disorder, 58

bacteria. *See* microbiota
bacterial amyloids, 140
Baltimore, David, 177
basal ganglia, 68
BE FAST mnemonic, 112
behavioral variant, 98, 106
benzodiazepines, 260
bioflavonoids, 240–2
bismuth, 268
blood–brain barrier, 18, 32
bovine spongiform
    encephalopathy (BSE),
    118–21, 143
brain, 42–54, 59
  aging and, 15
  alcohol and the, 124
  Alzheimer's and, 28, 84–6, 90
  attention and, 294
  blood–brain barrier, 18, 32
  gut–brain pathway, 89, 142–5
  inflammation and, 17, 18
  interconnections, 62
  learning and, 201–3
  microbiota and, 47, 58–9, 74
  neuroimaging, 92
  organ systems and, 152–8
  sensitivity to injury, 109
  structure and learning, 30–2
brain damage, 52, 53

brain-derived neurotrophic factor
    (BDNF), 33
brain hemorrhages, 85
Buddhism, 211

C9ORF72 mutation, 179
cardiovascular disease, 188, 201,
    225, 230, 233
celiac disease, 228
cerebellum, 68
cerebral amyloid angiopathy, 112
cerebral hemispheres, 57, 62
cerebrospinal fluid, 117
cerebrovascular diseases, 108–9,
    112
chess, 202
cholinesterase inhibitors, 95
chronic obstructive pulmonary
    disease, 157
chronic traumatic
    encephalopathy (CTE), 121–3,
    270
clinical syndrome, 76
clinical trials, 266–8
Clostridiodes difficile, 146
co-evolution, 134
cognition, 60–75
cognitive activities, 16, 30. *See also*
    mental activity
cognitive impairment, 41, 63, 78,
    259
  mild, 80
  rapid onset of, 41
  vascular, 111, 112
cognitive reserve, 16, 25, 26–32,
    59
  adaptability, 45
  dementia and, 32
  sleep and, 222
cognitive reserve capacity, 65
collaterals, 110

colon cancer, 138, 226, 268
colonization, 131–2
comorbidities, 41, 159
compliance, 260
consciousness, 50
corpus callosum, 62
cortical atrophy, 85, 86
cortical basal degeneration, 124
cortisol, 220
Covid-19, 153, 264
Creutzfeldt–Jakob Disease,
    118–21
crystallized intelligence, 75
curcumin, 241

Darwin, Charles, 123
delirium, 80, 148
delusions, 75, 80, 82
dementia, 76, 98, 104–6. *See also*
    Alzheimer's disease
  case studies, 106, 112
  cognitive reserve and, 32
  consultants for, 93
  music and, 68
  treatable and reversible, 96,
    106, 117
denial, 212–15
depression, 34, 70, 96, 161–9
despair, 35
Deter, Auguste, 82
diabetes, 112, 154, 198, 232
diagnostic tests, 287–9
diazepam, 106, 260
diet, 225–45. *See also* microbiota
  diverse, 133, 227
  gene therapy, 137–9
  inflammation and, 17
  natural foods, 236
  plant-based, 230
  public policy and, 283

recommendations, 245
disinhibition, 98
diversity, 41, 132, 195, 202, 227,
    267
DNA, 171, 285
dog ownership, 217
Down syndrome, 85
driving, 269
dysbiosis, 154

early-onset Alzheimer's disease,
    174
education, 26, 78, 99, 282
Einstein, Albert, 106
embolism, 107, 110
Emerson, Ralph, 60, 67, 296
encephalitis, 153
encoding, 67, 69, 203
endocrine system, 154
engram, 56
epilepsy, 58
episodic memory, 68
evolution, 19–24, 134
executive functioning, 79
exercise. *See* physical activity
experience, 56, 203
explicit denial, 213

falls, 148, 269
family history, 256
fasting, 242–3
fecal microbiota transplant, 146
fiber, 136, 138, 146, 227–9
fish, 226, 231
fitness, 8. *See also* physical
    activity
flavonoids, 236, 240–2
folic acid, 92, 237, 238
football, 121, 270
forgetfulness, 72–4, 106, 203, 207

frailty, 133, 149, 157
Frankl, Viktor, 34, 161, 209, 292
free radicals, 17, 85, 90, 235
frontal lobes, 57
frontotemporal lobar
    degeneration (FTLD), 96–9,
    106, 178, 180
fruit flies (*Drosophila melanogaster*),
    268
functional capacity, 65

gait disturbance, 117
Gajdusek, Daniel Carleton, 118
Gardner, Martin, 62
gastrointestinal tract, 153
gene–environment interactions,
    172–4, 178
genes, 171, 179
    amyotrophic lateral sclerosis,
        104
    APOE gene, 170–1, 174–81
    FTLD, 99
    gene therapy, 137–9
    Parkinson's disease, 101, 102
genetic mutations, 174
genetic testing, 171–81, 284–5
genomics, 284
Glenner, George, 85
glucocorticoids, 220
glucose, 53, 109
glutamate receptor blockers, 95
green tea, 241
Gulliver's Travels (Swift), 8
gut microbes. *See* microbiota
gut–brain pathway, 89, 142–5

hallucinations, 63, 80
head injuries, 121–3, 270–2
head, movement of the, 51
healthspan vs. lifespan, 9

hearing problems, 156, 204
heart disease. *See* cardiovascular
    disease
hemorrhage, 85, 107, 110
herpes viruses, 132, 264
hip fracture, 148, 269
hippocampus, 48, 68, 189
HIV/AIDS, 124, 266
holobiont, 285
homeostasis, 9, 153
homocysteine, 238
hunter–gatherers, 19, 133, 225,
    228
hydration, 243
hyoscyamine, 106
hypertension, 94, 111, 112, 156,
    157, 187, 242

immune response, 139, 149, 153
immune system, 16–19, 89
immunity
    adaptive, 17, 88, 139
    innate, 16, 88, 139
    microbiota and, 139
implicit denial, 213
infarct, 108, 110
infections, 131–2, 153
inflammaging, 17
inflammation, 16, 33, 139, 246
    Alzheimer's, 88
    anti- and pro-states, 17, 18
    APOE gene, 176
    brain and, 17, 18
    microbiota and, 17
innate immunity, 16, 88, 139
integrity, 35
intelligence, 61, 75
interdependence
    brain and body, 42
    interactions, 148–52

ionic gradient, 53
ions, 53

Jackson, John Hughlings, 52
James, William, 70, 169, 203, 209, 211, 292, 294
Juno space probe, 49

Katzman, Robert, 26, 84
kidney disease, 33, 158
Kraepelin, Emil, 82
kuru, 118, 143

lactobacillus, 246
language learning, 47
lead poisoning, 275
learning, 30–2, 47, 201–3
Lewy body disease, 101–3, 222
life expectancy, 11, 20, 83, 281
lifespan vs. healthspan, 9
lifestyle behaviors, 90, 164
Lister, Joseph, 240
liver, 158, 276
London taxi drivers, 47
loneliness, 37

macrophages, 58
magnesium, 239, 240
magnetic resonance imaging, 3, 92, 106
Man's Search for Meaning (Frankl), 161, 209
maternal affection, 189, 220
McGregor, Dr. Alyson, 83
meaning, search for, 34, 209–10
medications, 254–5, 259–63
    personalized, 284–5
    research registries and trials, 266–8
meditation, 210–11, 294

Mediterranean diet, 230
Melville, Herman, 64
memory, 60–75
    components of, 203
    drugs and supplements for, 263
    sleep and, 222
    stress and, 219
memory loss, 67, 70, 75, 76, 79
memory strategies, 207
memory trace, 56, 67
meningitis, 153
mental activity, 23, 27, 200–5. *See also* learning
mental status examination, 92
mercury, 275
metagenome, 127
metagenomics, 285–7
metaphors, 45
Metchnikoff, Elie, 246
microbial DNA, 285
microbiome, 127
microbiota, 16, 126–33, 134, 153, 246–8. *See also* diet
    brain and, 47, 58–9, 74
    diet and, 137–9
    disease around the world, 135–7
    disease treatments, 145–7
    diverse, 132, 227
    gut–brain pathway, 89, 142–5
    immunity and, 139
    inflammation and, 17
    influence on the body, 133
    metagenomics, 285–7
    neurodegeneration and, 140–2
    oral, 133–4, 249
    Parkinson's disease, 103
    physical reserve and, 32
    stroke and, 112
microglia, 47, 58, 73

mild cognitive impairment, 80
Miller, Daniel, 48
minerals, 238, 240
misfolded proteins, 19, 143
Moby Dick (Melville), 64
motor neuron disease. *See*
      amyotrophic lateral sclerosis
      (ALS)
multiple reserves, 113
   Alzheimer's disease and, 39
   delaying onset of dementia, 105
   public policy and, 282
   whole body health, 198
multiple system atrophy, 124
multivitamins, 239
muscle mass, 14
music, 13, 48, 68, 202, 209
myelin sheath, 15

Natural History of the Intellect
      (Emerson), 60, 67
natural selection, 19
Nesse, Randolph, 167
neural networks, 51
neurodegeneration, 18. *See also*
      dementia
   diagnosis, 287–9
   microbiota and, 140–2
neurofibrillary tangles, 28, 82,
      85
neuroimaging of the brain, 92
neuronal firing, 31
neuronal networks, 30
neuronal reserve. *See* cognitive
      reserve
neurons, 49, 54, 56–7, 88
neurosyphilis, 81, 82
neurotransmitters, 49, 260
Newton, Sir Isaac, 62
niches, 154

normal pressure hydrocephalus,
      117
Nun Study of Aging and
      Alzheimer's Disease, 29

obesity, 155, 198, 214, 232
oligosaccharides, 126
omega-3 polyunsaturated fatty
      acids, 231
opportunity of aging, 5, 11, 296
oral health, 133, 134, 159, 249
organ systems
   brain health and, 152–8
   physical exercise and, 194
organs, 42–4
osteoporosis, 149, 269
otolith organs, 51
oxidative stress, 222
oxidative toxicity, 85
oxygen supply, 53, 109

pain, 159, 196
Parkinson's disease, 37, 101–3,
      105, 144, 222
Pasteur, Louis, 265
pathogens, xiii, 135
perception, 74
periodontitis, 112, 133, 159
personalized medicine, 284–5
pesticides, 274, 283
phages, 146
phenylketonuria, 173
physical activity, 33, 192–7
   depression and, 168
   stroke and, 112
physical reserve, 16, 25, 32–4, 199
   interdependent factors, 148–52
physicians, 250–4, 257, 258
phytoestrogens, 241
Piaget, Jean, 66

Pick's disease. *See* frontotemporal
    lobar degeneration (FTLD)
plasticity of the brain, 46, 47–51
pneumonia, 148, 153
polypharmacy, 96, 259, 291
polyphenols, 240–2, 286
positron emission tomography
    (PET), 86, 106, 287
post-traumatic stress disorder
    (PTSD), 166, 219, 220
prebiotics, 146, 248, 286
Prevagen, 263
primary progressive aphasia, 98
prion disorders, 118, 120, 143
prions, 87
probiotics, 146, 246, 247, 286
procedural memory, 68
progressive supranuclear palsy,
    123
pro-inflammatory state, 17, 18
proteins, 86
    folding, 87–8
    misfolded, 19, 143
Prusiner, Stanley, 140
psychological reserve, 25, 34–6
    management of, 206–8
public policy, 41, 282–3

quality of life, 8

Reagan, President Ronald, 212
recent memory, 66, 67, 75, 79
red meat, 226, 229
remote memory, 66
research, 264–5
research registries, 266–8
reserve capacities, 8, 10
reserve factors, 25–41
resilience, 8, 65. *See also* cognitive
    reserve
resistance, 89

retrieval, 67, 203
risk factors
    Alzheimer's, 93, 188
    Parkinson's disease, 102
    stroke, 111
Roosevelt, Franklin Delano, 66

salt, 225, 242
salutogenesis, 9
saturated fat, 136, 225, 226
scrapie, 118
semantic dementia, 98
semicircular canals, 51
sensory cortex, 57
sensory deficits, 156
sensory functions, 63
shingles, 132
short-chain fatty acids, 139
sleep, 222–4
smartphones, 289
smoking, 33, 102, 187, 274
snacking, 235
social contacts, 216–18
social isolation, 36, 166
social media, 164
social networks, 36, 37, 167
social reserve, 25, 36–8
spinal column, 272
storage, 67, 203
stories, 204
stress response, 189
stress, coping with, 34, 219–21
stroke, 107–8, 109, 110–12, 188
    diet and, 225, 230
sugar, 232–5
surgery, response to, 148, 159,
    160
Swift, Jonathan, 8
symbiosis, 126, 128
synapses, 49, 58
syphilis of the nervous system, 124

systemic reserve. *See* physical
    reserve
systemic toxic-metabolic
    conditions, 96

tau, 85, 86
television, 164, 200–1
temporal arteritis, 258
temporal lobes, 57, 62, 68
tennis, 26, 48, 192
thrombosis, 107, 110
time, passage of, 293
tolerance, 89
toxic exposures, 199, 268, 274–7
toxins, protection from, 158
tranquilizers, 168
trauma, 270–3
TREM2 gene, 178
trimethylamine, 112, 154, 231,
    286
trimethylamine oxide, 154, 231

underweight, 149, 155
urinary tract infections, 42

vaccinations, 263
vagus nerve, 143

vascular cognitive impairment,
    111, 112
viruses, 128, 132, 146, 264
visual cortex, 47, 57
visual hallucinations, 63
visual problems, 156, 258
vitamin B12, 92, 148, 238, 240
vitamin B6, 92, 237, 238
vitamin D, 149, 239
vitamins, 237–40

water balance, 243
Wernicke Korsakoff syndrome,
    124
whole-genome sequencing, 284
wisdom, 75
women
    Alzheimer's disease and, 78
    life expectancy, 83
    loneliness and, 37
working memory, 69
worldwide aging, 281

yogurt, 246, 247

zidovudine, 266
zinc, 238